Food Power: Nutrition and Your Child's Behavior

Also by James Presley
Center of the Storm: Memoirs of John T. Scopes
Please, Doctor, Do Something!
Vitamin B_6, The Doctor's Report
Public Defender
Human Life Styling

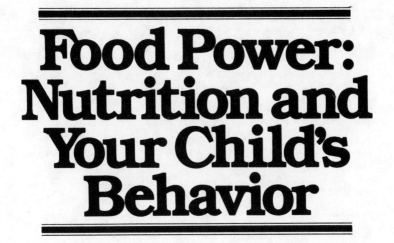

Food Power: Nutrition and Your Child's Behavior

Hugh Powers, M.D.
James Presley

St. Martin's Press
New York

Library of Congress Cataloging in Publication Data

Powers, Hugh.
    Food power.

    1.   Children—Nutrition.   2.   Children—
Nutrition—Psycholgical aspects.   3.   Emotional
problems of children—Nutritional aspects.
I.   Presley, James, joint author.   II.   Title.
RJ206.P68   618.9′28′90654   77-15919
ISBN 0-312-29776-9

For the many grateful patients
helped through improved nutrition.

—H.P.

For Fran and our children, John and Ann
Presley, who became active partners in
the writing of this book.

—J.P.

In order to protect privacy, all patient's names used herein have been changed.

Contents

1

Mood-Changing Foods

To be studiously tactful and kind, you might say Mary Sue was "temperamental." But to be painfully truthful, you would be forced to admit she was a holy terror—aggressive, hostile, and hyperactive.

Almost ten, she continually tormented, teased, and struck her playmates. At home she wandered restlessly from room to room, handling forbidden, fragile articles, and throwing objects. In school she had a short attention span, wouldn't finish her work, dawdled, and talked endlessly. Her penmanship, never very good, deteriorated. She was a fourth-grader, doing third-grade work.

Mary Sue's health was poor. She'd had asthma and her legs ached. Every several days, she complained, she felt "funny things" in her right leg. Her appetite was wretched; instead of eating, she talked constantly at mealtimes.

Mary Sue's problems can be divided into three major categories:
1. Behavior
2. Learning
3. General health.

Her behavior, most of all, had driven her parents, teachers, and playmates to despair. Everything from medical remedies to psychology had been tried, and nothing had worked. At this point, more out of desperation than optimism, Mary Sue was brought to me. I am a specialist in orthomolecular pediatrics. Orthomolecular therapy means supplying the body with those substances natural to it but which, for some reason, it has not been getting or absorbing. Basically, this means nutritional programming.

Most of us realize how important nutrition is to a child's growth and how it provides energy for playing and studying. But we sometimes overlook other ways in which food is crucial to the child's health and well-being. It may influence how he feels toward the world and the people around him. (For convenience, "he" will be used hereafter when "he or she" is meant.) His moods may be intimately affected by his nutrition. What he eats and drinks may play a major role in whether he is pleasant or hostile. Some foods and beverages spell Trouble for some children, and may be damaging to all children even when the effects aren't obvious. They should be avoided. Other foods are healthy, encourage pleasant moods, and should be on the menu for all children.

This book is about nutrition and what you can do to insure that your child benefits from the proper foods and escapes the consequences of the wrong ones.

In Mary Sue's case, as in all such cases, it was necessary to first rule out the possibility of a disease affecting a specific organ. Although she had already had medical attention, in order to insure that some disorder had not been overlooked, I gave her a thorough physical examination. Poor coördination of her right hand and arm indicated the possibility of brain damage, but there was no evidence from any of the tests that Mary Sue was suffering from a specific disease that might account for her behavior. After talking with her mother, I compiled a detailed picture of Mary Sue's daily nutritional pattern, and her diet revealed the direction of the treatment.

BREAKFAST

Refined cereal with *sugar*
White toast with *jelly,* or with cinnamon and *sugar*
An egg occasionally
Milk

MORNING SNACK

Doughnut or *cookie*
Or cheese and *white crackers*
Milk

LUNCH

Hot lunch or hamburger with *white buns*
Milk
Corn chips, cookies, or carrots
Fruit pudding and/or *cake*
Tea twice a day

AFTERNOON SNACK

Corn chips or *potato chips*
Apple
Cookies
Cola drink occasionally

3

Milk
Cheese and *crackers*

DINNER

Ham or hamburger usually as meat dish

No seconds except for *refined spaghetti*, milk, *cake, chocolate cookies*, or fruit *pie*

The suspicious foods in Mary Sue's diet are italicized. They are all capable of creating a metabolic imbalance called carbohydrate overload. Refined sugar and refined starches are mood-changing foods to which many growing children are especially sensitive. Usually the impact can be ascertained by comparing the child's diet with his behavior. But to pin it down precisely, laboratory tests may be necessary. The most effective test for diagnosing the dangers of carbohydrate overload is the glucose tolerance test (GTT), which tells us how the body is handling carbohydrate foods and whether blood sugar (glucose) levels are stable.

For the GTT, the patient reports to the laboratory in the morning before eating breakfast. A fasting blood sample is taken. Then the patient swallows a specially sweetened liquid on an empty stomach. Blood samples, and sometimes urine samples, are taken at regular intervals for the duration of the five-hour test. This offers objective lab evidence of how well the patient is maintaining glucose (blood sugar) in the bloodstream, which eventually conveys it to the brain. Glucose is an essential fuel for the brain and, therefore, is essential to the whole body.

The ideal standard for such a test (based on the work of Dr. John W. Tintera) is shown by the fine-line graph in Figure 1-1. Let's compare it with Mary Sue's test, which is depicted by the heavy line.

Figure 1-1. Mary Sue's Glucose Tolerance Test

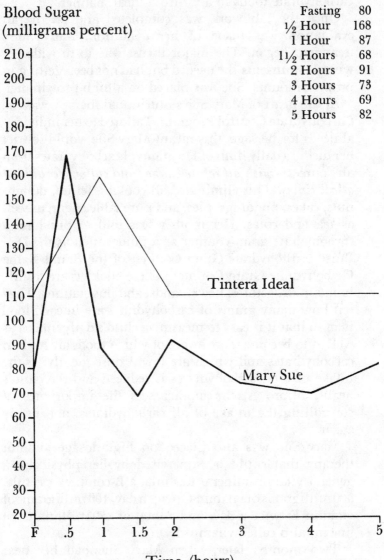

Blood Sugar
(milligrams percent)

Fasting	80
½ Hour	168
1 Hour	87
1½ Hours	68
2 Hours	91
3 Hours	73
4 Hours	69
5 Hours	82

Tintera Ideal

Mary Sue

Time (hours)

Mary Sue was suffering from a *carbohydrate overload* and her body was handling her sugar and other carbohydrate foods in a far-from-ideal manner.

Once the lab work was completed and an overall evaluation was made of her condition, Mary Sue's treatment began. The major thrust was to provide her with the nutrients she needed but had not been getting in proper amounts. She was placed on a high protein diet.

At the heart of Mary Sue's nutritional therapy was the Carbohydrate Control Program. Tailored to her individual needs for her age, this meant Mary Sue would restrict her diet to a daily limit of 115 grams of carbohydrates from all sources—*with all refined sugar and caffein forbidden at all times*. This eliminated all cookies, jellies, doughnuts, cakes, puddings, pies, and pure table sugar, as well as tea and colas. Her mother was told to purchase a carbohydrate gram counter as a guide, such as the Dell Purse Carbohydrate Gram Counter of the Brand Name Carbohydrate Gram Counter. These booklets are readily found in drugstores, news stands, and bus stations. They tell how many grams of carbohydrates are in each food item so that it is easy to measure a child's daily intake, as well as to become more aware of which foods are high in carbohydrates and which are low. Consequently, as the intake of total carbohydrates is reduced and the child's health improves, the mother sees the importance of controlling the intake of all carbohydrates, not merely sugar.

Mary Sue was also placed on high-dosage vitamin therapy that could be supervised by her physician: a general vitamin-mineral formula, a B-complex capsule, 500 milligrams of vitamin C twice a day, 100 milligrams of vitamin E twice a day, and a total of 250 milligrams of niacin (also called vitamin B_3).

Two months later, when Mary Sue had her next

appointment, she had changed remarkably. She was by no means perfect, but her mother reported Mary Sue was much more relaxed. Mary Sue's teacher said the little girl was now easier to work with and had a longer attention span. The poor writing persisted, but she had no leg pains, was pleased with herself for a change, and behaved well with other children. During her examination she was a quiet, informative, and *sweet* child, improved in nearly every way.

Her mood-changing foods had been eliminated and Mary Sue herself recognized the difference when she said, "I'm not as bad as I used to be."

At this point, because Mary Sue was a growing child, her overall carbohydrate intake was increased slightly, to 125 grams daily. All sugars and refined starches remained forbidden. There were no changes in the type of food she could eat but only in the amount.

Three and a half months later, at a followup exam, Mary Sue was better in *all* respects. Now she finished her homework alone and her handwriting had improved. Her mother was advised to increase the carbohydrate limit to 135 grams daily, while continuing to exclude sugar and caffein.

Orthomolecular Pediatrics—in this case, a combination of carbohydrate control, high protein diet, and vitamin therapy—had brought about remarkable changes in Mary Sue. The approach that improved her behavior can be expected to work on most other children, including those with quite different specific problems of behavior, learning, and health. The key is the carbohydrate control program, which is one that benefits *all* children. Seemingly normal children who are suffering from carbohydrate overload may not react with any of Mary Sue's symptoms, but at the very least they are probably not enjoying their highest possible level of health. Symptoms may not materialize for months or years in some children. If the parents control the carbohydrates early enough, the symptoms may never appear.

Mary Sue had what might be termed a "typical" recovery. Her program was a standard one that is used as a starting point. With the vast majority of patients, it works. With some, results come almost immediately; with others, it takes longer than it did with Mary Sue. At times, it may become necessary to modify the basic program, if the child fails to improve after a fair period of time. Some children, I have observed, are made nervous by high dosages of the B vitamins. The doctor then halts everything and approaches the problem from a new direction. It may not have been a vitamin-mineral deficiency, after all, but something to do with the specific food intake. Other children, however, may need specific vitamins in *massive* doses. This was true of one hyperactive child, who required extremely high supplementation of niacin and vitamin C. Occasionally, a hair sample analysis may be required, to determine if there is a toxic buildup of heavy metals such as mercury, and a doctor's attention, of course, is necessary in these cases.

But the most common affliction of the children discussed in this book is carbohydrate overload. Until this excess is elminated, it is futile to expect any complete recovery for Mary Sue and the millions like her today. Sugar and other easily absorbed carbohydrates and stimulants must be removed from the diet, and a limit must be placed even on the acceptable carbohydrates, so as to insure a balance of food types. Once this is done, most children change for the better in every way.

Blood Sugar and the GTT

In recent years, much has been written about low blood

sugar. Most physicians do not diagnose low blood sugar until the level has dropped to 30 or 40 milligrams percent, and very few of the patients in this book experienced drops to that classical low. Therefore, this book is not about low blood sugar—it is concerned with the *instability* of blood sugar and those foods containing unacceptable carbohydrates that play havoc with blood sugar levels and cause mood instability in children. It should be emphasized that a blood sugar problem is not a disease itself but a symptom like fever that shows something is wrong in the body.

The specific problem can usually be pinpointed by a glucose tolerance test, or GTT. Traditionally the GTT is used to diagnose either diabetes, which is high blood sugar, or hypoglycemia, which is low blood sugar. In diabetes, the blood sugar level soars above all normal heights and tends to remain there. In low blood sugar, the level sometimes drops low enough to cause blackouts or faint feelings; in some cases, it starts low and stays low.

What my patient Mary Sue suffered from, however, was an unstable blood sugar level. It dropped lower than it should have; more significantly, it went up and down in a jagged, abnormal fashion. When a child's blood sugar acts in such a bizarre manner, with *rapid* changes, there is no way to insure a smooth-operating nervous system. The child will not feel well, will not behave well, and will not be well.

There are three basic groups of abnormal blood sugar curves afflicting children today. They can be characterized by the type of symptoms which each one tends to produce, and are illustrated in figures 1.2, 1.3, and 1.4.

Although these patterns are different, the goal of treatment should be the same: to stabilize the blood sugar so that the children's bodies and especially their brains— which require more blood sugar than any other organ— will operate smoothly and efficiently.

Pediatricians and Blood Sugar

The standard pediatric approach does not include an examination of the child's blood sugar patterns unless some extreme medical problem is suspected, such as diabetes or exceedingly low blood sugar. All too often, little or no attention is given the child's nutritional status past the period of very early childhood when baby's formula and baby foods are discussed. Very soon, drugs become the main means of treating the various disorders of childhood.

Unfortunately, a constellation of highly-promoted new "wonder" drugs has failed to provide the stable blood sugar that children need. Otherwise, the runny noses, stomach aches, disruptive behavior, and learning disabilities of children might now be decreasing rather than increasing. No one knows this better than the pediatrician who faces the daily frustration of dealing with forty to seventy patients, many of whom have been sick all winter with hardly a respite.

I learned this from my own pediatric practice before shifting my approach to that of orthomolecular pediatrics. I had worked overtime trying to vanquish the symptoms of colds and infections; all measures seemed to be but temporary stopgaps, however, as the patients inevitably returned with similar illnesses.

My interest in this new approach developed slowly from one of drug treatment that merely relieved the symptoms. I first became interested in the multiple problems of the nervous system and their effects upon learning. Why didn't these children's brains work better? Along with Dr. James R. Hill, a colleague who specializes in internal medicine, I turned to the glucose tolerance test as a diagnostic tool. The use of blood sugar evaluations wasn't new; it traced back to Dr. Seale Harris in the 1920s. I

Figure 1-2. Sample Blood Sugar Curve Depicting Irritability

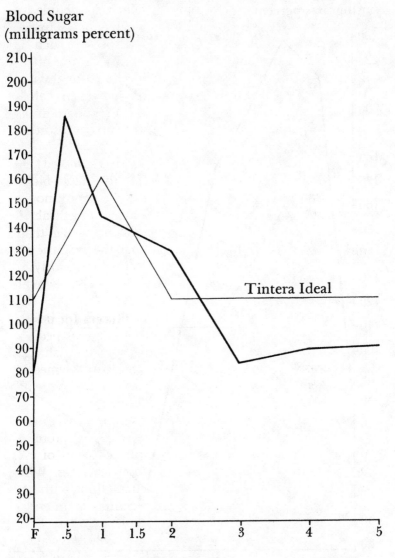

Blood Sugar
(milligrams percent)

Tintera Ideal

Time (hours)

This type of blood sugar curve was too high for too long before decreasing in a kind of "stair–step" pattern. For the last few hours it is usually lower than it should be. This curve indicates abrupt changes in blood sugar which would make anyone irritable.

Figure 1-3. Sample Blood Sugar Curve Depicting Psychosomatic Symptoms

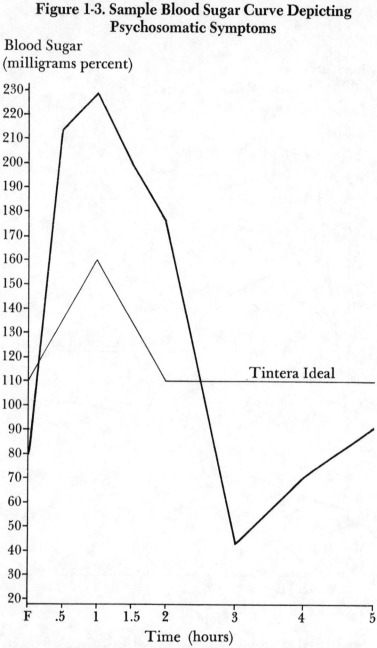

Blood Sugar
(milligrams percent)

Tintera Ideal

Time (hours)

This type of blood sugar curve climbed high and then dropped very suddenly to unusually low levels. In the fourth and fifth hours of testing, the child's blood sugar climbs upward but is not back to the "ideal" level by the time the test has ended. This often produces psychosomatic symptoms.

Figure 1-4. Sample Blood Sugar Curve Depicting Listlessness

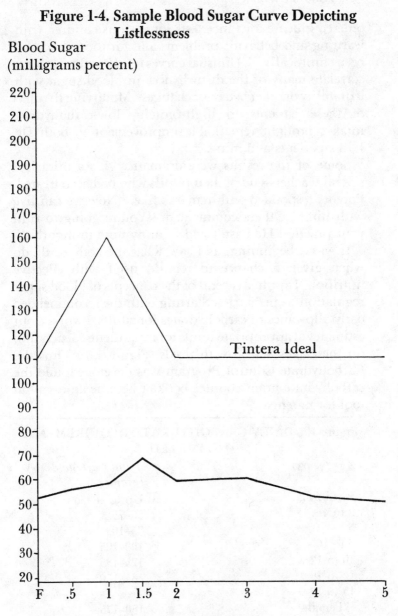

Blood Sugar
(milligrams percent)

Tintera Ideal

Time (hours)

This type of blood sugar curve neither rose nor fell. The fasting level is much lower than normal. When the glucose drink is swallowed at the beginning of the test, the curve rises only a little and remains low thereafter. These so–called "flat" curves are associated with listlessness and moodiness.

ordered glucose tolerance tests for various children with learning and behavior problems and for those who had been chronically ill. Unusual curves resulted. I was able to correlate many of the disturbances in blood sugar with irritability or other behavior changes. Modifying the diets of these patients to high-protein, low-carbohydrate intakes brought remarkable improvement to both Dr. Hill's patients and mine.

Some of the results were dramatic. "It's a miracle," several teachers said of their pupils who had been treated. Parents responded with remarks like, "Now we can live with him!" Others commented, "You're going to ruin your practice. He hasn't had a runny nose in months."

It was a beginning, as I saw what the body could do when given a chance to rebuild itself with effective nutrition. I applied several of the concepts of blood sugar regulation to pediatrics. Starting with the recommended daily allowance of carbohydrates for adults, I worked out estimates of appropriate limits for my patients, depending on their ages and growth needs (Figure 1.5). Thus the Carbohydrate Control Program was developed, and the carbohydrate gram counter booklet became an essential tool for parents.

Figure 1.5. DAILY CARBOHYDRATE REQUIREMENTS (ESTIMATED)

Age (years)	Total Carbohydrates (grams)
Birth to 2	Up to 40–50
2 to 4	50–75
5	75–100
6 to 10	100–125
10 to 12	125–135
12 to 15	135–150
15 to 18	
Female	150–175
Male	Up to 200–250

I must emphasize that these are *estimates* of carbohydrate limits, based upon my own clinical observations. Nobody has yet determined the exact carbohydrate requirements of the growing child. These estimates are keyed to the body's recognized energy needs, based on 150 calories per kilogram (2.2 pounds) of body weight. It is never possible to work realistically with the human body on the basis of inflexible numbers. A child's needs may vary, depending on size and appetite, and it is therefore important to use this chart as a guide only.

As I worked more and more with my patients, it became apparent that their general health, as well as behavior and learning, was vastly improved through nutrition. If the child was involved in any phase of a special educational program, he did better when it was combined with a sound nutritional regimen. The child who had virtually lived in the doctor's office came in less and less often; he simply wasn't falling prey to the usual onslaught of infections.

Then came other cases, ones that other physicians could not help or had lost interest in or said could not be improved. With a nutritional program, these children did do better. Each new case inspired confidence and enthusiasm beyond expectation.

The Carbohydrate Control Program was extended to all my patients, whether they had sharply disturbing symptoms or not. If they had handicaps in school or had severe brain damage and were on physical training programs, they all improved significantly when the carbohydrate intake was monitored and modified. It soon became evident that this nutritional approach was one that would benefit *all* children, from babies to teenagers—even into adult life.

It is necessary to emphasize, however, that elimination of the easily absorbed *refined* carbohydrates should not lead the parent to cut down on the *complex* carbohydrates which are essential to growth and weight gain. With those children in whom my basic program may not produce the expected results, recent evidence indicates that blood sugar may also be stabilized with a low fat, low cholesterol, moderate protein, and relatively high complex carbohydrate diet. Such a modification would involve using breads, crackers, and cereals made from *unrefined* flour at meals and serving *lean* protein snacks.

Linus Pauling and Orthomolecular Psychiatry

Dr. Linus Pauling, Nobel laureate in Chemistry and in Peace, is responsible for popularizing the term, orthomolecular psychiatry, which is not as awesome as it sounds. Simply stated, orthomolecular psychiatry means the treatment of mental disorders by providing the nutrients that the brain and nervous system need in order to operate at top efficiency. The emphasis is on those substances which are "normally present in the human body" but which, for various reasons, are not available to be utilized by the brain.

There may be many reasons why the brain cells are not receiving what they need. There could be a genetic factor that short-circuits the processing of food within the body or creates a larger-than-normal demand for a particular substance. Or the individual may not be eating the food he needs; he could be eating the wrong kind of food. And, as Dr. Pauling pointed out, in today's rapidly changing world, we may not always have the best selection.

Brain and nerve tissues are the most sensitive of human tissue, as far as the rate of chemical reactions is concerned. Dr. Pauling believes this is why the mental symptoms of certain vitamin deficiency diseases sometime occur before physical ones. Among the substances that have been helpful in treating schizophrenia, a leading mental

16

disease today, have been vitamin C and three of the B vitamins—vitamin B_6, vitamin B_{12}, and nicotinic acid (B_3). For some reason, these patients weren't receiving enough of these vitamins or weren't utilizing them as their bodies required for normal functioning. Vitamin C and the B vitamins are necessary for the body's normal chemical processes, and when they are used to help the patient's body and mind function as they should, it is a case of orthomolecular psychiatry in action.

Drugs, however, are not normally found in the human system. Whether extracted from plants or synthesized, they are alien substances to our bodies. For this reason, there is always a risk when you introduce one into your system—although there may be occasions, of course, when their use is necessary. The orthomolecular approach to disease therapy and prevention primarily involves nutrition. Except for the occasional injection of a vitamin, mineral, or hormone, we absorb these substances through the process of digestion. This means that the molecules of life are supplied by our food and food supplements: vitamins, minerals, protein, carbohydrates, fats—all the nutrients that our bodies need.

Dr. Pauling himself summed up the theme of orthomolecular medicine:

"Having the right molecules in the right amounts in the right place in the human body at the right time is a necessary condition for good health."

This book will apply the principles of orthomolecular medicine and psychiatry to the treatment and prevention of various childhood disorders. If children have the right molecules in the right place at the right time, they are likely to enjoy better health and to have control over their behavior. With their minds functioning normally, they can enhance their learning ability.

Every day we deliver molecules to our brains and other

parts of our bodies through nutrition. Whether we know it or not, we are influencing our mental and physical conditions. The same is true for our children. By concentrating on nutritional elements that are apt to provide the right molecules for growing children, we are following the principles of orthomolecular pediatrics. And if your child doesn't seem to have any problems, you can use the program to *prevent* a breakdown of health, whether your child is still a baby or already a teenager.

Graphically we can depict the importance of nutrition in your child's life with the cycle of health shown in Figure 1-6. At the top of the cycle is the healthy, happy child. At the bottom is the unhealthy child whose inadequate nutrition has left him vulnerable to the stresses of modern life. A major function of this book will be to explain how to keep your child at the top of the cycle.

Eight Ways to Evaluate the Quality of Your Child's Medical Care

In order to determine if your child is benefiting from his or her medical care, here are some questions you might want to ask yourself:

1. Is there an excessive reliance on drugs, as opposed to rehabilitation or prevention programs?

2. Do there seem to be too many, or too great a variety or frequency of, infections?

3. Have appropriate tests been made to ferret out the major medical causes of an illness? These might include blood tests for anemia, examining for organ diseases (such as urinary obstruction, etc.), or a thorough survey of chest sinuses and mastoids. Consultations with specialists might be advisable in some instances. Have allergy investigations been made in cases justifying it?

4. Is your child's home environment psychologically sound? If your doctor hasn't inquired into this, you might

Figure 1-6

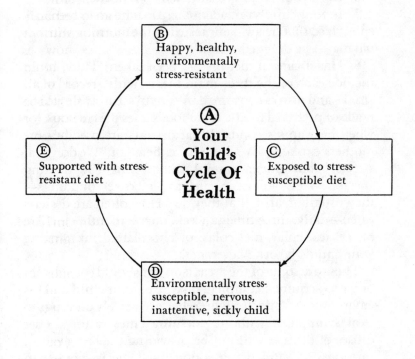

Ⓑ Happy, healthy, environmentally stress-resistant

Ⓐ Your Child's Cycle Of Health

Ⓔ Supported with stress-resistant diet

Ⓒ Exposed to stress-susceptible diet

Ⓓ Environmentally stress-susceptible, nervous, inattentive, sickly child

– Corbett Anderson

consider it as objectively as you can.

5. Is your child overworked? Activities that might contribute to an overload, in the susceptible child, include an early paper route, football practice, piano and ballet practice, and Brownie troop meetings on top of an already crowded schedule. A review of the child's weekly obligations might be revealing.

6. Does your child get sufficient physical exercise?

7. Is your child's rest adequate? Does he go to bed early enough so that he awakens rested in the morning without having to be dragged out of bed?

8. Has a careful diet history been taken? This should include each of the three main meals, with a record of all snacks and drinks consumed. A careful scrutiny should be made of preferred foods. What foods does the child ask for when he wants seconds? What desserts are used? (Some mothers explain, "We don't have them" or "We don't eat sweets," but under careful questioning—by naming specific sweets or desserts, such as pies, cakes, puddings— they usually realize that they do.) How often are desserts eaten—daily, three times a week, once a month, etc.? Are coffee, tea, colas, diet colas, or chocolate drinks among your child's favorite beverages?

These are some of the areas a doctor should consider, in order to acquire a complete picture of your child and his environment. A doctor who relies excessively on drugs to treat symptoms, without pursuing clues to the deeper causes of disease, will not be providing the best medical care possible. Practicing sound medicine is more than looking at a sore throat or a nervous child and writing a prescription.

But even when your doctor is nutrition oriented, the role of the parent remains extremely important. In order to really evaluate a child's health, the parent must be aware of how food affects the body. In the next chapter we will look at food and nutrition in depth.

2

Fuel for Human Machinery

Glucose and the Brain

Food is the prime fuel for human machinery. Without the precise fuel that it has been designed to use, supplied in the right amounts so that that there is a steady flow, the machine will not run properly. Ironically, this probably is appreciated better by those who own pets or who make their living from raising animals such as cattle, sheep, and horses. In most cases, the science of nutrition is applied more thoughtfully to those animals than to their human owners. More care is given frequently to feeding a dog or a cat than to the child who plays with it. Who would feed a pet poodle cake, sugary colas, pizzas, and doughnuts?

If we compare the human body with an intricate machine, we can say that it consists of other, smaller machines. The heart, for instance, is a pump. The lungs are a breathing machine, the kidneys a complicated apparatus for elimination. The brain, a chemical machine made of living cells, is the one particularly relevant to learning and behavior, and it is equally pertinent to general health. Although every "machine" in the body plays a role in health, the brain is probably the most sensitive to changes in body chemistry. For this reason, a child's food intake is of utmost importance, for what goes into his digestive system is going to influence his brain. If vital substances are left out of the diet, complex disruptions may occur in the brain that will affect the rest of the body.

Glucose, a simple sugar, is the main source of energy for the brain. But the glucose used is the end product of an amazingly complex series of biochemical transformations that begin with digestion. In breaking down food, the digestive system processes the raw materials that our bodies utilize. Eventually the blood stream conveys the glucose to the brain, where it is used as energy. For the brain to function at top efficiency it must have an even, steady flow of glucose.

As the "machine'" most affected by the availability of glucose, the brain requires a stable blood sugar to ensure a reliable, smooth supply of energy. If there is not enough, the mind falters. If there is a sudden rush of glucose, as might happen when a caffeinated or sweetened drink is ingested, the brain becomes overcharged. Either way, there is stress upon the brain which affects the rest of the body. This is why a major emphasis should be placed upon carbohydrate control and the stabilization of blood sugar in a child. Sugar abuses directly affect the operation of the child's brain, which in turn influence how well he is to learn and how he will behave. These are the readily seen results, but deterioration of the child's general health is a slower, less dramatic process that often goes unrecognized.

Effective learning, acceptable behavior, and good

health are direct results of a healthy and efficient brain. To reach this goal, it is necessary to eliminate carbohydrate *abuse* and insure that the child's nutrition is sound and complete. With that done, a high grade fuel (glucose), flowing steadily to the brain as it should, is practically guaranteed. An approximate analogy is that of the gasoline engine: if the carburetor feeds in too much gasoline, the engine is flooded; if it doesn't receive enough, the engine is "starved" and sputters. Roughly, we can say the same of glucose as energy for the brain.

High-Grade Human Fuel

There are eight groups of ingredients that mix together to produce a high-grade human fuel: protein, fat, carbohydrate, vitamins, minerals, trace elements, water, and oxygen. When the blend is perfect, the result is a spectacular improvement in an individual's health and well-being. Let's take each of them in turn.

CARBOHYDRATES. We have said that a carbohydrate overload can cause disturbing symptoms in children. But what is a carbohydrate food? Composed of a combination of carbon, hydrogen, and oxygen, carbohydrates are the cheapest and the fastest digested of the three major food substances. Carbohydrate is found in fruits, vegetables, juices, grains, sugars, and milk. Nature seems to want to impress us with the vital aspect of carbohydrates, for the brain uses more of it, in the form of glucose, than any other tissue or organ. When the supply of carbohydrates is not adequate, exhaustion occurs, and growth in children ceases.

The major types of carbohydrates are sugars and starches. Starches can be broken down in the body to form sugars. The best sources of starches are vegetables and grains, such as potatoes, legumes, breads, and cereals.

Bread, the product of wheat, corn, barley, or other grains, is a leading form of starch in the American diet. Although sugars are found in a variety of foods ranging from vegetables to milk, they mostly come from fruit, certain vegetables, and special foods like honey. Table sugar comes from the refining of beets and cane.

The term, *refined* carbohydrates, usually refers to carbohydrate foodstuffs that have been through the milling process, during which much of the original raw material has been removed. In the case of flour used to make white bread, this means the wheat berry has undergone serious surgery; the wheat germ, a rich source of vitamin E and the B vitamins, and the outer bran, containing minerals and valuable fiber or bulk, are both removed. The endosperm of the wheat berry is left. It is practically all starch. The grain of wheat has been "scalped." In the case of white bread, three synthetic B vitamins and iron are "returned" to the loaf as part of what is called the "enriching" process.

The same, but more drastic, fate befalls sugar cane that is used to produce white sugar. When the sugar cane stalk is processed, all of its fiber, its vitamins, and its minerals are removed. The molasses vanishes. Only the refined, white sugar crystals remain. This sucrose, as table sugar is called, is, in effect, a drug, containing only *refined* carbohydrates and calories. It is extremely concentrated and is often added to packaged cereal products, which themselves are refined starches.

Why are these foods processed to this point? The reason, basically, is economic. If the natural, whole food were left with its active ingredients, it might sprout or even decay. Refrigeration would be required to keep it fresh. This would necessitate more expense to the food merchant. But through a procedure of intensive milling, the food company can insure a long "shelf life" for the product. The active ingredients have been taken out, but the remaining refined carbohydrates are not the same raw material the human body has been handling for hundreds of thousands of years: the body is left with a surfeit of concentrated starch and sugar, which it is not equipped to handle on a steady basis.

On the other hand, the unrefined or natural carbohydrates of vegetables and fruits provide other food elements, such as vitamins and minerals and sometimes fats and proteins. A raw peach, for example, is a natural carbohydrate food; in addition to its total carbohydrate (sugar) content, it provides a small amount of protein, a little fat, a plentiful supply of vitamin A, and varying degrees of calcium, phosphorus, iron, potassium, B vitamins, and vitamin C. It also has enzymes that are needed for the proper metabolism of that food.

The difference between a refined and a natural carbohydrate is seen when we compare brown, unrefined rice with white, polished rice. The natural brown rice has more protein, fat, calcium, phosphorus (twice as much), potassium (twice as much), and niacin. An equal amount of white, polished rice has more total carbohydrates (starches) because that is mainly what is left after milling. In other words, the milling process strips out a significant percentage of nutrients, and although some such milled products are then "enriched," there is never as much added as was taken away. The brown rice, and other natural carbohydrates, not only supply a complex of recognized nutrients, but it seems likely they may also contain unknown nutritional factors as yet undetermined.

Generally speaking, approximately half of one's calories should come from natural, or complex, carbohydrates.

Let's compare two short lists, one of refined sugars and starches, the other of natural carbohydrate-containing foods.

25

Natural Carbohydrates	Refined Carbohydrates
Apple (raw)	Table sugar
Whole-grain bread	White bread
Banana	Ice cream
Squash	Cola, soda pop
Brown, unpolished rice	Spaghetti from refined flour
Sweet potato	Pie, cake

An easy way to distinguish the two types of carbohydrates is to remember that the natural foods are whole, the refined ones have been tampered with and are incomplete.

PROTEIN.   Protein is the master food substance of the body. It is present in every cell, tissue, and enzyme in the body, in one form or another. It is involved in hormones, muscle contraction, and immunological responses. In experimental studies with rats, protein deficiency has caused slower development and mental retardation; protein and caloric malnutrition has led to poor mental development in children.

Protein provides the building blocks of growth in a child. The body also uses protein for repair. This means it is required twenty-four hours a day. The growing child especially needs a stable, steady supply of it.

Protein is extra important during the three major periods of rapid growth in a child's life: at infancy when he or she is gaining about two pounds a month, at the minor growth period beginning around ages five and six, and during puberty and adolescence.

There are two types of protein, the animal-source protein and the vegetable-source protein. The human body tends to operate most efficiently with animal protein or with a mixture of both animal and vegetable protein.

When eaten together, animal protein enhances the vegetable protein.

Protein is made up of amino acids; thus, their reputation as the building blocks of protein. The human organism uses twenty amino acids, and all but eight can be synthesized in the body. Those eight are therefore classified as "essential" to the human being and must come from food. In order to insure a supply of the essential amino acids daily, I recommend a daily supply of animal-source protein, such as a serving of meat, fish, egg, fowl, or cheese at each meal. If for some reason animal protein cannot be supplied three times a day, it should be balanced with vegetable protein such as that in legumes like peas and soybeans.

The chart in Figure 2.1 will provide a general guide for calories and protein requirements of children at different ages. The size of the servings would depend on the size, age, and appetite of the child.

Many packaged cereals claim to contain protein. However, such cereals vary in protein content and are of relatively low quality. The highest quality protein is in the outer layers of the seed and around the embryo or germ of the grains and is usually removed by milling. Thus, complete cereals like rolled oats, unpolished rice, and wheat germ are generally healthier.

In order to maintain a good supply of protein, all we need to know are the foods in which protein is found. The best animal sources of protein are eggs, fish, chicken, beef, and pork; milk and cheese also rate high.

In the plant world, the protein leaders are soybeans, beans, peas, and nuts. Foods containing vegetable or plant protein also contain carbohydrates and sometimes fat.

Figure 2.1. PROTEIN AND TOTAL CALORIE
REQUIREMENTS OF THE GROWING CHILD*

Age (yrs.)	Weight (lbs.)	Height (ins.)	Protein (gms.)	Calories
Birth–2 mos.	9	22	kg x 2.2	kg x 120
2 mos–6 mos.	15	25	kg x 2.0	kg x 110
6 mos–1	20	28	kg x 1.8	kg x 100
1–2	26	32	25	1100
2–3	31	36	25	1250
3–4	35	39	30	1400
4–6	42	43	30	1600
6–8	51	48	35	2000
8–10	62	52	40	2200
10–12,				
Males	77	55	45	2500
Females	77	56	50	2250
12–14,				
Males	95	59	50	2700
Females	97	61	50	2300
14–18, Males	130	67	60	3000
14–16, Females	114	62	55	2400
16–18, Females	119	63	55	2300

*Recommended daily allowances (Revised 1968), Food and Nutrition Board, National Academy of Sciences-National Research Council.

FATS. Fats—the right kind—are essential to health. There are many kinds, but we can simplify the situation by dividing the fats into two groups: the saturated and the unsaturated. *Unsaturated* fats remain liquid at room temperature; these are the right kinds for health. *Saturated* fats congeal and harden at room temperature; these are to be avoided in the diet.

The *essential fatty acids,* found in unsaturated fats, are

the ones we need every day in our diet. The body requires linoleic and linolenic acids; if it has these, it can synthesize another required fatty acid, arachidonic acid. Vitamin B_6 seems to be required to convert linoleic acid to arachidonic acid. The best sources of linoleic and linolenic acids are sunflower seed, corn, safflower, and soybean oils.

As long ago as 1929, experimental work with rats indicated the essential fatty acids were necessary for growth and well-being. It is likely that all animal species, including humans, need a small amount of these essential fatty acids each day. They have a major role in the manufacture of prostaglandins, important hormones that are found throughout the body. Prostaglandins are thought to be biological factors in controlling blood pressure, in smooth muscle contraction, and bringing about synthesis of enzymes and hormones.

Dietary fat can be converted by the liver into acetate, which is necessary for the utilization of blood sugar energy in the brain cells. An insufficient supply of acetate can eventually lower the energy output of the nervous system. Elimination of fats from the diet would be disastrous, for the essential fatty acids make a contribution to the health of every cell in the body.

The minimum daily requirements of fat in the diet are not known, but fat probably should provide at least 10 percent of the calories in the diet and not more than 35 percent.

Recent evidence compiled by the Longevity Foundation of America, at Santa Barbara, California, and other researchers indicates that fats may be as much of a culprit as sugar in the American diet. In addition to a long–accepted role for cholesterol in cardiovascular disease, fat may be a factor in diabetes in that high fat levels in the blood may decrease the efficiency of insulin. Drs. James W. Anderson of the San Francisco Veterans

Administration Hospital and Robert H. Herman of the U.S. Army Medical Research and Nutrition Laboratory at Fitzsimons General Hospital in Denver have shown that increased fats in the blood may contribute to irregular blood sugars. Drs. Anderson and Herman have introduced, for most of their hypoglycemia patients, a low fat, high complex carbohydrate diet in which 45 percent of the calories come from these complex carbohydrates. They avoid the rapidly absorbed sugars.

Although some researchers believe that the adult diet should not contain more than 5 to 10 percent fats, the requirements of the child may be different. The precise requirements for children are not yet known, but fats are particularly essential for the process of myelination, the formation of the myelin sheaths of nerve fibers. Because of these very significant needs, the fat content should never drop below 10 percent in the child's diet, but should never compose more than 35 percent. As we will see, most diets would automatically supply 10 percent or more fats in the diet.

While polyunsaturated oils, from vegetable sources, contribute to health, the role of the saturated fats is suspect. These are mostly of animal origin and have been indicted by many researchers as factors in cardiovascular disease. To saturated fats of animal origin, such as lard and meat grease, hydrogenated oils must be added. The process of hydrogenation changes unsaturated oils into saturated fats; the oils are hardened by adding a catalyst which is then heated to saturate the oil's carbon atoms with hydrogen. This is done for the commercial motive of keeping the oil from spoiling—to insure a longer shelf life. But once an oil is hydrogenated, it is no longer an unsaturated vegetable oil that can be recommended for health. It should be avoided along with hard animal fats. Saturated fats are factors in raising the blood cholesterol level. The cholesterol count can be lowered by replacing animal and hydrogenated fats with polyunsaturated fats of vegetable origin. However, there probably is little need for added fats in most diets, as properly balanced meals will automatically provide the requirements. Frying of any food is discouraged, but use light butter or a margarine that hasn't been hydrogenated, if frying must be done; excessive heating of polyunsaturated oils brings about changes in those fats that may make them carcinogenic (cancer causing). The best rule to follow is to always use polyunsaturates, *unheated,* as in salads. If you must use fats in cooking, use butter or olive oil.

Beef, mutton, poultry, and fish are good protein foods which contain saturated fats; purchase lean cuts and organ meats and trim off the excess fat. Cheese and butter have saturated fats but are permissible as long as not too much is consumed and they are balanced with other foods. Although some pork organ cuts may be acceptable, most muscle pork is higher in fats than other meat; bacon is not only mostly hard fat, it also contains probable carcinogenic preservatives. The main goal is to keep the saturated fats in the diet as low as possible, with unsaturated fats taking their place.

Good sources of unsaturated fats are margarine, peanut butter, and salad and cooking oils. However, most commercial brands of margarine and peanut butter have been hydrogenated. It is important to read the labels to make sure the products have not been hydrogenated or "hardened." Organic versions of these foods, sold in health food stores and sometimes in other groceries, are unsaturated. If they are organic and unhydrogenated, the labels are practically certain to say so, for the company will be aware of the difference and will be proud to advertise the fact.

Although most vegetable oils are likely to be unsaturat-

31

ed and sources of essential fatty acids, there are exceptions. Coconut oil contains mostly saturated fats, with very little essential fatty acids. It should be avoided, along with hydrogenated fats.

VITAMINS. Basically, there are two types of vitamins, and your child needs both. They are the *fat-soluble* and the *water-soluble* vitamins. Fat-soluble means they can be stored in the liver and used another day. Water-soluble means that daily excesses are passed in the urine. This means that each day the child must have a new supply of the water-soluble vitamins, regardless of the quantity consumed the day before.

The fat-soluble vitamins are A, D, E, and K, and the water-soluble vitamins are C and those of the B-complex.

By consulting the chart (Figure 2.2) you will have an idea of your child's vitamin needs. The Recommended Daily Allowance is probably closer to minimum requirements for health than to maximum needs. Individuals will vary and children may require more than these recommended allowances.

Vitamin E is known to improve utilization of vitamin A. Because E conserves oxygen, it may be presumed to enhance cerebral function. In fact, I have observed this clinically in children with learning disabilities. Good sources of vitamin E are wheat germ and vegetable oils.

Vitamin K is the blood-clotting factor found in certain green vegetables and it is necessary to health, although less is known about it than the other vitamins.

Vitamin A is essential to healthy eyes and skin and is helpful in preventing infections. A total absence of vitamin A has been found in some individuals in certain primitive cultures. The pitiful victims suffered from a condition known as xerophthalmia, a drying and disintegration of the cornea, which can lead to blindness and total destruction of the eye. This illustrates the extreme to which the deficiency may go, but a mild deficiency of vitamin A causes a slight drying of the skin and swelling of the hair follicles—symptoms which may be overlooked by many parents.

A medium-sized sweet potato, baked in its skin, will provide around 8000 units of vitamin A, for instance. A small serving of beef liver will supply the daily needs for vitamin A, even though the values in cuts of liver may vary widely. Other good sources of the vitamin are carrots (10,000 units for 3½ ounces, cooked) and cantaloupe (½ small provides 6000 units). Mustard greens, spinach, and collard greens also supply generous quantities of vitamin A.

Vitamin D is required primarily for good bone structure. In the small child, a deficiency may result in rickets. Vitamin D can be formed on the skin from sunshine, provided the skin has sufficient natural oils and is not washed for several hours afterward so as to remove the vitamin. The best sources are fish liver oil, rather than synthetic vitamin D, known as irradiated ergosterol.

A question frequently asked by mothers, regarding vitamin supplementation, is, "Doctor, can my child get too much?" The answer is that with the fat-soluble vitamins A and D, it is possible to overdo it. Unlike the water-soluble vitamins, excesses of vitamins A and D are not readily excreted in the urine. Therefore, they may store up in the liver and if the dosages are extremely high, toxic effects may result. For this reason vitamin A supplements should be limited to 5000 to 10,000 units per day for a child. Excessive accumulation of vitamin A through *very* high dosages may cause symptoms that mimic brain disorders, to mention a more serious side effect, along with blurred vision, headaches, or loss of hair.

Vitamin D supplementation should be kept within 400

to 800 units daily. Overdoses of vitamin D may disturb the delicate balance of calcium, magnesium, and phosphorus in the body.

It is important to remember, however, that when I discuss overdoses of vitamins A and D, I am referring to vitamin supplements—not food. You do not have to worry about your child's getting too much vitamin A and vitamin D from food in a normal diet.

With the water-soluble vitamins—the B-complex and C vitamins—the question of toxicity is a different matter, for no harmful effects have been demonstrated when high dosages are given. Although some individuals have exhibited temporary overload reactions to extremely high dosages—rashes and diarrhea from vitamin C, and excitement, headaches, or sleeplessness from the B complex—the overwhelming concern with these vitamins should be with the possibility of deficiencies.

The functions of the B-complex family are varied. This group works with minerals to activate enzyme systems in the body. (An enzyme is a cell-secreted protein that causes chemical changes in other substances without itself being affected; it is a catalyst in thousands of bodily reactions, including digestion.) Vitamins B_1 (thiamin), B_2 (riboflavin), and B_3 (niacin) help steady nerves, improve appetite and digestion, and contribute to good morale. A serious lack of them can cause beriberi and pellagra.

The blatant signs of vitamin deficiency diseases stand out and can be spotted. For instance, pellagra, caused by an absence in the diet of niacin, or vitamin B_3, brings on the "three D's": dementia (general mental deterioration), dermatitis, and diarrhea. On the other hand, partial deficiency states are difficult to recognize in apparently well-fed people. For example, inadequate amounts of B-complex vitamins are associated with irritability and fatigue, which in turn may easily be confused with irritability and fatigue from other causes, such as an allergy. It is well to remember that a child does not jump from a well-nourished, healthy state to one in which there is a total deficiency of a vitamin or mineral. The child is more likely to move *gradually toward* a deficiency condition and over a period of years suffer from a partial deficiency without being aware of it. And, as is usually the case, he will suffer from a lack of several nutrients, rather than merely one.

Figure 2.2. VITAMINS*

Age (yrs.)	Fat-Soluble				Water-Soluble					
	A	D	E	B₁	B₂	Nia-cin	B₆	B₁₂	Folic Acid	C
	(IU)	(IU)	(IU)	(mg)	(mg)	(mg)	(mg)	(mcg)	(mcg)	(mg)
Birth–6 mos.	1400	400	4	0.3	0.4	5	0.3	0.3	50	35
6 mos.–1	2000	400	5	0.5	0.6	8	0.4	0.3	50	35
1–3	2000	400	7	0.7	0.8	9	0.6	1.0	100	40
4–6	2500	400	9	0.9	1.1	12	0.9	1.5	200	40
7–10	3300	400	10	1.2	1.2	16	1.2	2.0	300	40
11–14										
Male	5000	400	12	1.4	1.5	18	1.6	3.0	400	45
Female	4000	400	10	1.2	1.3	16	1.6	3.0	400	45

*Daily allowances recommended by the Food and Nutrition Board, The National Academy of Sciences, National Research Council.

These recommendations, which are the "official" ones, are apt to be on the low side for a number of reasons that I will discuss. They can be used as a general guide when the child has no unusual problems. A supplementary table which may be useful in special cases is provided on page 41.

Borderline cases of B-complex deficiency are most commonly seen in this country. The best illustrations of this are the chronic grouch, the "lazy bones," the nervous child, and the teen ager with vague complaints. All of them may improve with vitamin B-complex supplementation. As co-enzymes, the B vitamins help convert foods into energy. Folic acid and vitamin B_{12} are vital to maintaining a healthy state of the blood. The best sources of folic acid are in a variety of fresh, unrefined foods as many of the B vitamins are widely distributed in nature.

Another B vitamin, pantothenic acid, is also widely distributed in foods in small amounts. It participates in the metabolism of fatty acids, plays a part in adrenal hormone synthesis, and is related to antibody (protein germ-fighters) formation, thereby helping the body develop an immunity to disease. The richest sources of pantothenic acid are liver, kidney, fresh vegetables, other organ meats, fresh grain cereals, yeast, and eggs.

In recent years we have become aware of the crucial metabolic role of vitamin B_6 (pyridoxine). It has been found to be necessary in more than seventy-five enzymatic reactions, some of them in the brain. Vitamin B_6 is essential for the proper functioning of protein-synthesizing enzymes and metabolism of the nervous system. Dr. John M. Ellis, a pioneering clinical authority on vitamin B_6, has linked its deficiency in adult patients to problems related to rheumatism, menstruation, diabetes, and heart disease. If inadequate amounts can so affect adults, it is logical to suspect that such partial deficiencies may have begun even as far back as childhood. This is one of the strongest reasons to begin early to correct such nutritional flaws, and it is why, in treating chronically sick children, I use a vitamin-mineral formula that provides 15 milligrams of vitamin B_6 a day instead of the "recommended daily allowances."

Other B vitamins have parallel essential roles. Vitamin B_{12} is necessary to form blood marrow cells. Biotin is the protein co-enzyme; it helps convert protein into energy, and is needed for growth. Choline, another B vitamin, contributes to aspects of fat metabolism and nerve function. These and other members of the B family are found in abundance in such foods as liver, brains, yeast, wheat germ, and eggs.

When individuals are under stress, their needs for the B vitamins are increased. One study found that persons who took large doses of pantothenic acid seemed better able to handle emotional stress—and were not harmed by the large quantities given them. Animal experiments have also shown increased learning ability when diets rich in the B vitamins are implemented.

Although most breads and cereals are artificially "enriched" with vitamins B_1, B_2, niacin, and protein factors, more has been taken away during the milling than was put back. They do not contain the complex of B vitamins as it was in the wheat grain in the beginning. For instance, the "enriching" process does not include vitamin B_6 and pantothenic acid. Instead of getting what he needs, the child receives an overload of starches and sugars and incomplete protein factors which may leave him worse off, in some ways, than before he ate. The average child is probably lacking in pantothenic acid. Many may approach a total absence of it; nausea, a symptom of such a deficiency, is fairly common among children today. It may be the reason many children shun breakfast. Other dietary deficiencies may be factors in disturbed sleep patterns, headaches, and leg cramps, which are too frequently shrugged off as "growing pains." In experimental work with rats, Dr. Roger J. Williams, a biochemist at the University of Texas at Austin, has shown that pantothenic acid-rich diets extended the life span of the experimental group over the control group by nearly 19 percent. He indicates that the addition of 20 to 25 milligrams of extra pantothenic acid, over a lifetime, might do the same for humans.

A wide variety of foods, as unprocessed as possible, is required for health. There are twenty-two foods tested as being high in vitamin B_6. If a child does not eat vegetables, he is likely to consume only 13 percent of the foods that will provide him with an adequate B_6 supply. The situation is made worse if the child consumes most of his food in the form of sugary cereals, pop tarts, sweet rolls, peanut-butter-and-jelly, and bread—without vegetables—and then tops it off with cake, pie, cookies, or ice cream. These high starch and sugar-filled snacks and meals not only deprive the child of essential vitamins and minerals, they also increase the need for B vitamins and other nutrients. In order to properly metabolize such refined carbohydrates, the body needs vitamins B_1, B_2, niacin, and pantothenic acid especially; the minerals magnesium and phosphorus are also required. Diets of highly refined starches and sugars are apt to be lacking or be very low in B vitamins essential to converting the food into fuel. Incomplete metabolism of these refined foods may leave waste materials like pyruvic acid and lactic acid that can lead to deterioration of the cells over a period of time.

As for vitamin C, another water-soluble vitamin, some very provocative discoveries have assigned it a major part in combatting the effects of stress upon the body. In one study with prison volunteers, severe emotional stress brought about a need for the vitamin that was three times that of normal conditions. This alone alerts us to the importance of increasing levels of this vitamin in helping to cope with various kinds of stress.

Vitamin C is used rapidly and in large quantities by the adrenal cortex. The adrenal cortex secretes an estimated thirty-two stress hormones, which are involved in the individual's sense of well-being and performance. Many children with poor eating habits face a long line of modern-day stresses: school and its constant demands, chronic infections, allergies, the psychic trauma of growing up in an increasingly complex, disjointed world, late hours, unstable and nerve-wracking changes in blood sugar levels, and various drugs, including the often unrecognized drugs such as nicotine, alcohol, and caffein. Along with changes in diet, vitamin C supplementation is usually necessary before they begin to feel and perform better.

Dr. Linus Pauling has demonstrated vitamin C's value against the common cold. Dr. Irwin Stone, naming it the "healing factor," has shown its protective role in the treatment of a variety of disorders ranging from viral and bacterial infection to cancer and wounds. In the clinic, Dr. Fred R. Klenner has been a leading pioneer in using high dosages of vitamin C in a number of disease conditions. It seems clear that we need more than the mimimum daily requirement (MDR)—which is the amount needed to avoid death or disability from scurvy.

Under normal conditions, a diet of natural, unrefined foods would provide adequate amounts of the water-soluble vitamins, preventing any danger of a complete deficiency. However, there are at least six situations that could lead to a subtle deficiency that might precipitate a more serious condition.

1. A lack of variety in foods.

2. A "top-heavy" diet that might cause specific nutrients to be lost or improperly utilized. By top-heavy I mean a diet that contains an excess of one element to the extent that it creates an unbalanced overload of that one element. For example, excessive consumption of milk, without the foods that supply sufficient magnesium, may bring too much phosphorus into the system to the detriment of the calcium-magnesium balance. An imbal-

ance between nutrients leads to displacement of other nutrients. For example, too much or too little of one of the B vitamins may leave the others less effective, and the absence of one essential amino acid (protein factor) may result in other amino acids' not being utilized.

3. Foods may be deficient in vitamins because of overrefinement.

4. Overheating through cooking may destroy certain vitamins. Many vegetables and all fruits should be eaten raw, and none overcooked.

5. Some foods spoil or deteriorate faster than others. Storing these foods for too long a time may damage their nutrient values.

6. Stress or disease, such as diarrhea, excessive emotional reactions, or lack of appetite, may waste or cause malabsorption of nutrients in the body itself.

Unfortunately, these situations occur more frequently than might be expected. The recommended daily allowance (RDA) of from 50 to 100 milligrams of vitamin C daily, about what an orange would produce, is insufficient to cover the exceptional needs of most children in today's stressful times.

There are no "official" tables of specific nutrient needs for infants, children, and adolescents for stress, depletion, or compensation for overrefined and under-reconstituted food. At this stage of knowledge there are only the individual physicians' empirical trial and error judgments based upon observations of the patients's response to supplementation. I use a scaled-down version of the adult vitamin and mineral levels that have been used in stress and orthomolecular work. This higher level of supplementation is used in at least three situations: if the GTT is associated with symptoms, if the diet history is high in refined "grain foods," sugars, and caffein, and/or if the child is under stress of school failure, behavior disorders, or sick a lot of the time.

Figure 2.3. APPROXIMATE VITAMIN NEEDS
FOR STRESS, POOR DIETS, AND
ERRATIC BLOOD SUGAR

Age (yrs.)	B_1, B_2, B_6 (mg)	Niacin (mg)	C (mg)	A (IU)	D (IU)
Birth–1	1.5	5	60	1200	400
1–5	10	25	150–600	1500	400
6–11	15	100	500–1500	3000	400
12–15	15	150–250	1000–3000	5000	800

Many physicians, aware of the effects of stress upon individuals, have begun applying megavitamin therapy with C and B vitamins in exceptional cases. To a child under five, a doctor might prescribe as much as 1000 milligrams (1 gram) of vitamin C, and consistently more for an older child or youth. In order to obtain an equivalent 1 gram of vitamin C from food, the child would have to eat about 13 medium-sized oranges or about three 6-ounce cans full of frozen orange juice concentrate. (Vitamin C tablets are best taken with food in order to prevent any possible acidic effect in the stomach.) While a deficiency of vitamin B_1 might be corrected with 1 to 2 milligrams a day, an anti-stress program might entail 15 to 25 milligrams daily or in older youths on a megavitamin program, 1 or 2 *grams* per day. Such large doses, of course, should be done under the supervision of the physician.

MINERALS. Minerals are activators of enzymes, which are catalysts in biochemical reactions. As such, minerals assist with innumerable vital functions in the body.

Those that are found in the body in large quantities are callled macrominerals. These include calcium, phosphorus, potassium, sulfur, sodium, chlorine, and magnesium.

41

A brief glance at some of their duties will give us a hint of what a deficiency may produce. Calcium's contribution to our bones and teeth is well known, but it is also essential to a healthy heart. The normal blood calcium/phosphorus ratio is 2:1 or 1:1 depending on age. Magnesium is also required for calcium balance; as such, it contributes to the smooth flow of nerve impulses. Magnesium, as we have already seen, is necessary for the metabolism of carbohydrates. Sodium is essential to fluid balance in the body. Potassium plays a part in metabolism of muscle and various organs, and chlorine is in gastric juices like hydrochloric acid which is essential to digestion, as well as a constitutent of the blood that is necessary to maintain the pH, or alkaline-acid balance.

OTHER MINERALS AND TRACE ELEMENTS. Iron is not found in quite the concentration as its companions, the macrominerals, but it is no less important. It is essential to hemoglobin formation, which is the red pigment in the red blood cells that carry life-giving oxygen to all parts of the body. Iron utilization is a complex process in the body, however, and oral supplementation with inorganic iron tablets is often ineffective. Other factors, such as protein, vitamin C, folic acid, and copper, also affect hemoglobin production.

Trace elements are found in relatively minute quantities in the body. Many are essential for metabolism and assist various hormones, enzymes, and even vitamins. Among the essential ones are iodine, zinc, manganese, copper, molybdenum, cobalt, and selenium. Selenium has now been shown to be a normal constituent of human milk. Copper is used by the body in many ways, including the metabolism or chemistry of nerve tissues. Zinc is known to be necessary for adequate growth, protein synthesis, and sexual maturation.

42

The essential biological minerals and trace elements are in a delicate reciprocal relationship with each other and must be in the proper balance. For example, excessive calcium intake can lead to zinc deficiency. Excessive zinc intake leads to iron deficiency anemia. Some investigators have even suggested that too much zinc in relation to copper may be a factor in coronary heart disease. An overabundance of manganese may bring on magnesium deficiency with its attendant nervous irritability and convulsions.

Because mineral and trace element interaction is so delicately balanced, the best safeguard against imbalance and the errors of quality would be a well-balanced diet of what Dr. Joe D. Nichols, the long-time president of Natural Food Associates, calls "natural, poison-free food grown on fertile soil, eaten fresh, and not overcooked." This enables the body to select what it needs from a wide range of high-quality raw materials. Happily, such foods are available. If you do not have your own organic garden so that you can grow your own food, most cities now have natural food stores that sell fresh produce grown without pesticides and synthetic fertilizers. In some places you may be able to buy directly from an organic farmer or a fruit-and-vegetable stand that advertises such food. Should organically-grown food not be available where you live, the next best thing would be to buy the freshest fruit and vegetables you can find. It is almost always possible to eat fresh food—and always possible not to overcook it.

The closer we can come to the natural state of nutrition—a totally unprocessed diet, fresh from the field or orchard or garden—the better off we and our children will be. At the same time it is realistic to acknowledge that we cannot always obtain perfect food. For this reason, many of us may need to supplement our diets with vitamins, minerals, and trace elements, plus protein reinforcement of some dietaries. Unfortunately, sufficient work has not been done to assure us of the precise requirements for the trace minerals, and when one mineral supplement is used by itself, there is a risk of creating an imbalance among the others. For this reason I find it necessary to emphasize that, first, food is the best source of minerals and, second, supplementation is best with a general all-around vitamin-mineral tablet or general mineral supplement that conveys all, or at least the major, minerals. Figure 2.4 will provide a general concept of the mineral needs of the growing child.

Figure 2.4. MINERAL REQUIREMENTS OF THE GROWING CHILD

Age (yrs)	Weight (lb)	Height (in)	Calcium (mg)	Iron (mg)	Magnesium (mg)	Phosphorus (mg)	Iodine (mcg)
Birth-6 mos.	15	25	500	10	60	400	40
6 mos-1	20	28	600	15	70	500	45
1-2	26	32	700	15	100	700	55
2-3	31	36	800	15	150	800	60
3-6	35-42	39-43	800	10	200	800	70-80
6-8	51	48	900	10	250	900	100
8-10	62	52	1000	10	250	1000	110
10-12							
Boys	77	55	1200	10	300	1200	125
Girls	77	56	1200	18	300	1200	110
12-14							
Boys	95	59	1400	18	350	1400	135
Girls	97	61	1300	18	350	1300	115

But even the vitamins and minerals do not conclude our list of substances that go into the fuel mixture for human machinery. There are two others, water and oxygen.

WATER. Since water transports all of the chemicals in the body, its concentration must be maintained within rigid limits to sustain life. For this reason, a person can go longer without food than he can without water before perishing.

OXYGEN. While not a food, but a gas, this final element in the fuel mixture is the indispensable constituent of all reactions in the body. Every cell in the body is dependent upon an adequate oxygen supply.

Regular exercise, especially that which improves heart and lung efficiency, not only helps keep the body at its peak, but also improves the effectiveness of oxygen intake and use. Running, walking, swimming, biking, and similar exercises are particularly helpful.

Obviously, oxygen utilization can be improved by not smoking. In addition to other risks, smoking depletes vitamin C and interferes with the transfer of oxygen from the lungs to the blood. Although smoking may have an impact anywhere in the body, it makes its first assault upon the breathing apparatus.

Adding all of these elements together, we can see that the support of the body's master tissue, the brain, as well as all of the other parts, requires a finely-balanced fuel made of the best food, plus sufficient water and oxygen. Neglect of *any one* of the elements in the energy mixture means a poorly-functioning chemical machine. It is even possible that much of what we think of as brain damage may be the result of a poorly-adjusted fuel supply.

The Four Food Groups

The first step toward insuring that your child receives adequate amounts of the eight basic nutritional elements we have just discussed is to feed him daily from the four

45

basic food groups. These are dairy products, animal and vegetable protein, vegetables and fruits, and whole-grain breads and cereals.

The best way to insure that a meal is balanced is to select one food from each group at every meal, although at least one meal should include two servings of the vegetable-fruit group. By balancing each meal, by varying the menus from day to day, and by avoiding sweets and overly refined foods, over a period of time your child is more likely to benefit from a balanced, wholesome diet.

DAIRY PRODUCTS. As well as being a major source of calcium and other minerals, dairy products provide protein, carbohydrates, and often fat. They are a reliable source of vitamin A and, to a lesser degree, members of the B complex.

Each of the following would constitute a serving: whole milk (8 ounces or 1 cup); skim, lowfat, or 2 percent milk (8 ounces); American or cheddar cheese (1½ ounces or 1½ slices); cottage cheese (1½ cups); and yogurt or buttermilk (8 ounces). A child over eight should have three servings daily from this group; a teenager, four servings. Portions are sometimes also used in cooking and thus are consumed through another food.

PROTEIN. Meat, eggs, and certain plant products constitute a major source of protein. They also contribute significant quantities of potassium, iron, and niacin. Organ cuts such as liver, kidney, and brain are even more endowed with iron and B vitamins.

For convenience I have included eggs and main sources of vegetable protein here. Each of these is a serving: meat—whether beef, pork, chicken, or fish (2 to 3 ounces, lean, cooked); eggs (2); organic peanut butter (4 tablespoons); dry beans or peas, cooked (1 cup); and nuts (½ cup). Everyone should have two of these daily; preferably they should have three servings.

Avoid hot dogs, bacon, and other meats that are high in fats as well as preservatives. Sodium nitrate which is used in preserving these meats has been indicted as a risk factor in bowel cancer.

VEGETABLES AND FRUITS. These foods are a major source of unrefined, whole carbohydrates, the kind the body needs, as well as some protein. Significant supplies of iron, calcium, phosphorus, and potassium are in vegetables and to some extent in fruit. Although a wide range of vitamins, minerals, and trace elements are in most fruits and vegetables, green, leafy vegetables tend to be abundantly endowed with vitamin A and potassium.

Servings: vegetable or fruit (½ cup); an apple, banana, orange, or potato (1 medium); grapefruit or cantaloupe (½ medium); juice of 1 lemon; orange or grapefruit juice (½ cup); fresh or fresh-frozen corn, peas, green beans, or beets (½ cup). These should include good sources of vitamins A and C. Vitamin C can be found in oranges, grapefruit, tomatoes, cantaloupes, strawberries (1 cup), broccoli (¾ cup), and raw cabbage (1½ cups). Broccoli, chard, all greens, kale, spinach, carrots, sweet potatoes, tomatoes, cantaloupes, and apricots are all high in vitamin A. Everyone should eat four servings from this group every day.

BREADS AND CEREALS. Whole-grain cereals and breads contribute vitamins E and B-complex, along with minerals and trace elements. Whole grains also provide fiber, or bulk, as do fruits and vegetables. Fiber is especially important to intestinal tone and is an aid to

47

preventing constipation and consequent disorders; white bread and highly refined cereals, on the other hand, may partially cause constipation.

A serving would consist of one of the following: one slice of whole-grain bread; cooked cereal (½ cup); macaroni or spaghetti from whole-grain flour or brown, unpolished rice (½ cup); 1 ounce (¾ cup) of dry whole-grain cereal; or six 2-inch square whole-grain type crackers. Four servings from this group are recommended for everyone.

Signs of a Poor Diet and Deficiencies

There are a number of signals your child may throw out that will tip you off to the fact that something is seriously wrong with his or her nutrition. Some of these may be signs, also, of a physical or psychological disorder, and in such cases the problem should be assessed by a skilled professional. However, in any case, the child's nutritional needs should be given attention. This review will explain the signs to look for.

1. *Irritability.* This is usually caused by a B-complex deficiency occurring with an excessive intake of refined breads, crackers, chips, and cereals with sugar and caffein.

2. *Poor sleep habits.* Usually a sign of excessive simple sugars (table and fruit), plus caffein in tea, coffee, and colas—all of which also create a relative deficiency of the B-complex.

3. *Fatigue.* Often a result of reactive or functional hypoglycemia (low blood sugar) from excessive sugars and caffeinated cola drinks.

4. *Inattention, poor concentration, loss of interest in school work, and failing grades.* B-complex deficiency and use of caffein and excess sugar.

5. *Frequent illnesses and prolonged recovery*. Relative deficiency of vitamin C when stress or any of the above exists. Frequent illnesses also may result from a lowered white blood count and decreased effectiveness of disease-fighting white cells, as the result of too much sugar, refined or natural.

6. *Sweet craving*. An excess of sweets and caffein. It may be relieved with a dietary prescription as presented throughout this book.

3

The Malnutrition
of Affluence

In the midst of affluence, children are filling their stomachs with junk foods to satisfy cravings, while starving their bodies. Satisfying a hunger for sweets is an abnormal event for human bodies. Yet within the past few decades it has come to be the accepted thing for children in this country. Affluent Americans have the money to buy the best of food; ironically, they frequently spend it for products low in nutritional quality—sugared drinks, "treats," and high-starch cereals and breads. Many children are slowly degenerating. Their cells are being deprived of valuable nutrients, which are being replaced by junk foods.

On the other hand, nourishing the body with high-efficiency food provides the daily requirements of all the nutrients through balanced selections from the four basic food groups. A positive force in metabolism begins, as each cell is supplied with what it needs. It is a choice of fuels that parents can make for their children, exchanging

50

a sputtering, incomplete one for a high octane mixture that makes for health.

The major concern of this chapter will be with the two primary factors in the malnutrition of affluence: protein starvation and sugar/refined carbohydrate abuse.

A typical case begins at about three years of age. The child has had one cold after another; none of the antibiotic drugs has slowed down the frequency. His teeth are decaying. Even the neighbors have noticed how tired and pale he is. Eventually the desperate parents pour out their frustrations to the pediatrician.

"We can't get him to eat a thing! We've done everything we know to try to make him eat. He's always sick. Just look at him! He's pale, has no energy and he's always fussing. Doctor, what *can* we do?"

A series of questions soon uncover a pattern now familiar to all pediatricians. Shortly after the child's first birthday, he began to display a progressive dislike for food. At first, both mother and father were mildly annoyed. Soon they became alarmed. They tried tonics, doubled vitamin doses, offered rewards, and played games at the table to encourage eating. Frustrated, the adults threatened, spanked, and made the child sit at the table for an hour, whether he ate or not. The nearest he came to eating was to hold a piece of meat in his mouth the entire hour, without devouring it, while drinking a glass of milk around the meat.

The mother gives the first clue to what the child is trying to survive on when she interjects, "He does drink tons of milk, Doctor!" At mealtimes he drinks only milk and consumes no solid food.

He's hungry soon after the regular mealtime and begs for snacks. By then the harried mother is ready to capitulate, anything to get some form of food into her child. Between meals, he fills up on white bread with jam, cookies, crackers, and candy, washed down with milk and soda.

A quick analysis of what these foods contain is the key to why the child is always sick, in poor humor, pale, tired, and unhappy. Milk has some protein but not enough; it is too dilute. Everything else he eats for the rest of the day is composed of refined carbohydrates. The child is suffering from protein starvation and sugar/refined carbohydrate abuse.

Protein Deficiency

Two earlier investigators of this particular form of protein deficiency, Drs. Harold D. Lynch and William D. Snively, Jr., have called it "a true deficiency disease" and one of the most prevalent conditions affecting children in the United States. This hypoproteinosis of childhood is quite common in families who spare no expense to feed their children. How could there be such cases of malnutrition in these better-off families? Lynch and Snively believed it is the result of "a general lack of understanding by parents of the fundamentals of nutrition."

They were describing a general condition that today affects millions of children on all social and economic levels. Many of them are suffering from protein deficiency; others are consuming enough protein quantitatively, but it is of low quality, as may be found in frankfurters. Eating high quality protein is no assurance children will get all the essential amino acids, if the meat is overcooked; excessive heat can destroy amino acids, though not as readily as it does vitamins. Even when properly-cooked meats and other protein foods are served, low-quality snack foods can cause a metabolic malfunction because the body is being deprived of other vital factors. Meat, after all, is not a complete food; your child still needs nutrients contributed by the plant kingdom. Not only is protein required, but the proper kinds of carbohydrates and fats are also necessary for that protein to be utilized efficiently.

Unfortunately, relatively few people in this country seem to be aware of the malnutrition of affluence. There has been no metabolic study of the physiology of good and bad diets or sufficient animal deficiency studies that would be comparable to the eating habits of millions of our children. Some work on specific deficiency has been done with rats. In one experiment, the mother was made zinc and manganese deficient and her offspring had abnormalities in the inner ear, ran screaming in circles, and swam in loops.

Four years ago I did a fifty-case computer analysis of patients' eating habits utilizing the services of the firm Dietronics, which demonstrated deficiencies in several nutrients in association with poor health and other problems. The British scientist John Yudkin's book *Sweet and Dangerous* documents the high risks of a sugar-laden diet. T.L. Cleave, G.D. Campbell, and N.S. Painter build an equally damning case in *Diabetes, Coronary Thrombosis, and the Saccharine Disease*. A number of other similar works have been published over the years. References frequently appear in *Prevention* and other magazines regarding how poorly nourished Americans are, even when prosperous.

Yet sufficient clinical evidence of the malnutrition of affluence awaits any pediatrician who is willing to spare the few minutes necessary to take a diet history of his patients.

The Misuse of Milk

Milk clearly has a place in children's diets, but it is far

from being the complete food that many believe it to be. In infancy it plays a major role in nutrition; by the age of two, its importance declines.

A number of myths have developed regarding milk: "The perfect food." "You never outgrow your need for milk." These catch-phrases are more of psychological than of physiological significance. Milk, which is 90 percent water, supplies an abundance of carbohydrates but is an inadequate source of other nutrients, such as the B-complex vitamins and iron. Fat is available in the form of cream in the milk, but the heavy milk-drinker often gets most of his vitamins in the form of supplements, which usually are doubled by his anxious parents.

Some protein is present in milk, but not enough. One ounce of milk provides only 1 gram of protein. Young children require from 40 to 50 grams of protein daily; a quart of milk would not be enough. It would require more milk than a small child could hold to insure the amount of protein necessary for muscle growth, the formation of blood, hormones, digestive juices, brain and nerve tissues, and disease-fighting antibodies, just to name a few of the many uses of protein by the body.

Past infancy, milk is merely a *supplemental* source of protein. From the age of two years on, the child must consume protein in the concentrated form found in meat, eggs, fish, or fowl. If he gulps large quantities of milk, accompanied by high-sugar, high-starch snacks, he spoils his appetite for other, growth-promoting foods.

Drs. Lynch and Snively reported a typical case of a nine-year-old boy who drank large quantities of milk and soft drinks, and ate cookies and crackers between meals. He refused meat and vegetables, had frequent vomiting, a poor appetite, and frequent stools. He was pale, poorly developed, and cavities were rampant.

Placed on a high-protein diet that excluded milk

altogether, with a small iron supplement, he gained weight in a month's time, recovered from his respiratory infections, and had a markedly improved appetite. Once the high-protein diet was a part of the child's daily routine, the voracious thirst for milk was curbed. At that point milk was prudently reintroduced into his diet.

Carbohydrate Overload and Sugar Abuse

What this child was not getting—and this is true of millions of children across America today—was the kind of food that would maintain his blood sugar at a stable level throughout the day, constantly supplying the brain with this energy in the *proper amount*. This stability of the blood sugar is called *homeostasis*, which signifies balance in the body. When the body is not in homeostasis, disease or catastrophe may not necessarily follow, but the brain will not function smoothly. Many neurological functions become rough and erratic, emotional outlook can become distorted, blood circulation may be affected; organ function and glandular output may become disturbed.

The brain is involved, either directly or indirectly, with all operations of the body. For instance, all muscle activity is related to nerve function, which is directly related to brain function and to the blood vessels. All intestinal and stomach muscles are involved. Thus, an erratic blood sugar level may cause muscular irregularities throughout the body, which would create unpleasant sensations, which in turn would be registered by the brain. This gives merely a hint of how important blood sugar levels are to the brain and, therefore, to the rest of the body.

Unstable blood sugar is inevitably involved in problems of health, behavior, and learning. This is frequently true even in cases where brain damage is also a contributing factor. In turn, the instability of blood sugar can almost always be traced to the single outstanding characteristic of the malnutrition of affluence: a refined carbohydrate overload.

The surfeit of refined carbohydrates will continue to be an obstacle to health even when the protein intake is sufficient. But in low protein diets, the role of refined carbohydrates is a particularly damaging one. In experimental work with pigs, B. S. Platt and associates reported in 1965 in the journal *Developmental Medicine and Child Neurology* that a significant addition of carbohydrates to a low-protein diet resulted in a worsening of already-bad health. Carbohydrate metabolism was deranged. Moreover, the low-protein diet *plus* added carbohydrates slowed brain activity to a greater degree than did the low-protein food alone.

Dr. John Yudkin, the British scientist who gave us the term, "malnutrition of affluence," and who has consistently been one of the world's most influential critics of sugar, has pointed out that rats consuming sugar have problems retaining and using the protein in their diets. In 1973 testimony before the Select Committee on Nutrition and Human Needs of the U.S. Senate, chaired by Senator George McGovern, Dr. Yudkin added: "In diets that are restricted in protein, the effect of the sucrose is to make the body lose protein more readily than diets without sucrose." He also made a number of other statements that must have startled Americans who have grown complacent with high sugar diets. "There is no physiological need for sucrose," Dr. Yudkin said. "The body reacts to this different metabolic behavior of sugar by a number of changes that, if produced by a food additive, would undoubtedly lead to its being banned." He continued, "I think the thing to do is to constantly stress that the body has no need for sugar at all." In other words, the body can manufacture all the glucose it needs from other materials, according to Dr. Yudkin.

Among some of the deleterious effects of refined sugar that have been demonstrated on either experimental animals or man were: diminished growth rate, decreased life span, production of experimental kwashiorkor (protein deficiency disease), increased deposition of body fat, increased blood concentration of cholesterol and of triglyceride (another fat that may be of more concern than cholesterol), impaired glucose tolerance ("chemical diabetes"), both increased and decreased blood concentration of insulin, increased liver size and liver fat, kidney enlargement, reduced pancreas size, pathological changes in the kidney, dental decay, induction of short-sightedness, increase of fat content in arteries, disturbed behavior of blood platelets, increase or decrease in several important enzymes in liver and in fat tissue, decreased ability to utilize dietary protein, and increase in the enzyme activity and the acidity of gastric juice.

Based upon Dr. Yudkin's work alone, the implications of carbohydrate overload in growing young humans are not comfortable to contemplate.

We have learned that carbohydrates consist of starches and sugars. A closer look will be helpful. Starches break down into sugars during the process of digestion. Basically, there are three forms of sugar: the monosaccharides, the disaccharides, and the polysaccharides.

The monosaccharides—the simple sugars—include glucose, fructose, and galactose. Fructose is fruit or grape sugar; glucose, the pure, simple form of sugar used by the brain, is found in fruits and vegetables. Each of these may combine with each other or other sugars to form a more complex sugar, as galactose does to become a constituent of lactose, the more complex sugar that is in milk.

The disaccharides break down to form two sugars.

Examples of disaccharides are maltose, lactose, and sucrose. Maltose is the product of starch breakdown and digestion; it contains two molecules of the simple sugar, glucose. Lactose, or milk sugar, is made up of a molecule each of the simple sugars galactose and glucose. Sucrose is composed of one molecule of fructose and one of glucose.

The polysaccharides, when broken down, consist of more than two simple sugars. The principal ones are found in the starches of breads, cereals, potatoes, and legume vegetables such as peas and beans.

On the basis of my medical observations with children, it appears that the simple sugars (fructose and glucose) and their combination in table sugar are the major culprits in disturbing the homeostasis, or stability, of blood sugar levels. This is particularly true when these sugars are consumed in large quantities or are taken by themselves, so that sugar literally floods into the blood stream. This causes a sudden elevation of blood sugar, but the pancreas responds, as if in panic, by releasing a flood of insulin to meet the emergency. Just as suddenly, the blood sugar is lowered. The end result is fatigue.

This should be sufficient to dispel the old myth about table sugar's value as energy. It is true that sugar represents calories—but nothing else—and that calories provide energy. A calorie, after all, is merely a unit by which we measure the heat-producing potential of food when it is oxidized in the body. However, the representation of sugar as an "energy food" is horribly misleading. *Your child does not need sugar to provide sufficient calories.* Any meal containing the right foods will automatically provide enough calories for energy, and because the body is breaking down more complex materials, there is no problem of sudden absorption, as there is with sugar. Another serious problem with refined sugar and starches is that, instead of energy, they may make extra *fat* in the body. Sucrose can also cause a disjointed metabolism. Instead of an energy food, table sugar is a *de*-energizing drug.

Furthermore, many substitutes for table sugar are just as bad. White sugar is pure sucrose, but raw sugar, brown sugar, and other so-called unrefined sugars are sucrose plus a few trace elements and in some instances contain soil residues. Although honey and molasses have certain nutrients in very small quantities that white sugar does not have, these will do the same to a child that white sugar will do, if he gets an equal amount. White table sugar, for instance, is 99.5 percent sucrose and 0.5 percent water. Raw sugar is 97 percent sucrose; brown sugar, 96.4 percent; maple sugar, 90 percent; honey, 82.3 percent; light molasses, 65 percent; and dark molasses, 55 percent. The rest is mostly water. Any one of these, of course, is an improvement of a sort over white sugar. The slight advantage of honey and molasses is that a person is not likely to eat as much as he would of pure white sugar. But children with a refined carbohydrate sensitivity may have the same reactions to raw honey's simple sugars, fructose, glucose, and sucrose.

Not only is sugar deleterious to a child's health and behavior, but even sucrose substitutes, I have observed, may trigger changes in behavior. Sorbitol is one of these. Found in mountain ash berries, sorbitol is used as a sweetening agent in many diet drinks, sugarless chewing gum, and the so-called sugarless diet cookies. It has caused irritability and fatigue in some of my patients. One boy, Frankie, was doing fine on his program until one day his mother offered him a "diet" cookie that contained sorbitol. Thirty minutes after eating it, Frankie was charging about the house. Sorbitol, a polysaccharide, is a readily utilized complex sugar and affects many people— those with unstable blood sugar—as readily as does sucrose. It whets the appetite for sweets and therefore should be avoided.

Saccharine, on the other hand, is a synthetic sweetener and has no apparent effect upon the blood sugar level. However, saccharine is similar to sorbitol in that it may cause a craving for real sweets.

What should be kept clearly in mind is that the absorption rate of sugars is of utmost importance. The body needs glucose, but it makes its own, available to the cells through the blood in a steady, well-regulated flow. The refined sugars are speedily absorbed, inundating the system, whether the source is table sugar or the sucrose of bottled drinks. The refined starches of white bread and pizzas are readily broken down into the simpler sugars. What the body needs is the sugar that is absorbed more slowly. This means the child should let his body process its own sugar from complex, unrefined carbohydrate foodstuffs, such as vegetables, fruits, and whole grain cereals and breads. This insures a slower rate of absorption, an apparently smoother utilization of the sugars thereby produced, and a much healthier child.

In feeding children, it is worth pointing out that many so-called health products contain quantities of sucrose and other sugars in the guise of these natural sweeteners. Even in many health food stores, candies and all varieties of sugary goodies are available. These are not made with white sugar but with honey, molasses, or raw sugar. The implication is that they are "healthy" because white sugar was not used. However, they must be assessed as sucrose sources.

Few parents probably realize what a tremendous increase in sugar consumption has occurred in this country. In 1815, it has been estimated, U.S. sugar consumption from all sources was 15 pounds per year per person. Today it is more than 120 pounds—a whopping

800 percent increase! Furthermore, those Americans under sixteen years of age probably now average from 140 to 150 pounds of sugar a year.

Obviously, these extra 125 to 135 pounds of sugar consumed each year are not needed for health or calories; it should be proof enough that a mere 15 pounds a year proved to be adequate back in 1815.

Today, sugar is added to almost everything, from baby's formula to even naturally-sweet foods such as bananas and sweet potatoes. The practice of adding sugar to formulas, which is totally unnecessary since lactose, a milk sugar, is found naturally in milk, has probably led to untold numbers of cases of sugar addiction or conditioning in the cradle, which is carried on into adult life. A major factor in this was the successful advertising of a corn syrup in the 1920s and 1930s, until it was widely recommended by doctors. Many a child has been brought up on Karo syrup and milk. The surface rationale behind this sugaring of milk was the child's prodigious growth rate during the first year of life—sometimes 18 pounds—compared to 4 pounds per year in the early school years. It seemed logical that this required extra calories and sugar was a concentrated form of calories. Such increased demands, however, can be met by the introduction of real foods when the baby needs more than breast milk or his formula.

If there is no valid reason to add sugar to a baby's formula, there is even less reason to add it to the food of an older child. At the age of two, the child enters a "plateau" period of slower growth until around the age of six, with reduced energy needs similar to the pre-puberty years. The important thing to remember is that (1) supplemental sugar does not convert into more energy and (2) it is detrimental during the growth periods and at all other times.

61

The youngster today is continually tempted by sugared food and drink. In each small glass of grape, orange, lemon, or lime soda, the child receives from 1 to 2 tablespoons of granulated sugar. Desserts may contribute much more. I took a personal survey of one soda fountain, heavily patronized by older children, and noted *fifty* posters plastered over a twenty-square-foot section, each advertising the "strawberry festival." This referred to five desserts filled with ice cream and various syrups. The queen of this sweet realm was the banana split: three sugar-laden scoops of ice cream, covered with at least two different kinds of syrups, whipped cream, nuts, maraschino cherries (which had been soaked in liquid sugar), and, like an afterthought, a banana.

These are merely a few more items that are a part of the nutritional wasteland in which, as far back as 1951, the sales of sweetened, carbonated beverages amounted to more than 25 *billion* dollars, the equivalent of $227 worth of soda pop for every person in this country. A single hint of the impact on the nation's health can be gained by pondering the comment of Nobel laureate Sir Frederick G. Banting of Canada, the co-discoverer of insulin for the treatment of diabetes:

"Hard soft-drinkers produce more cirrhosis of the liver than hard hard-drinkers."

Today, sugar permeates most children's lives. Sweets are given as treats and bribes. Psychologists sometimes seek to modify behavior by offering candies. Candy and soda pop machines are found even in the primary schools. How can a child be expected to be temperate when the adults everywhere force sugar upon him?

Few parents seem to be aware of the seriousness of this threat to their children's health. Part of the problem parents face is the cumulative effect of daily, intense pressures to feed their children an oversweet diet. The addition of sugar to commercial foodstuffs has reached the point where at times it seems impossible to find food that has not been adulterated with sugar.

Parental Ignorance

Feeding a child of any age is not easy. But we can all offer the right food and deny the wrong food for a start.

The problem is in recognizing what the right food is. Today the parent is assailed on every side by sales pitches and, frequently, blatantly false information. When it comes to nutrition, you can find an advocate for any view or any pseudo-food. It is not surprising that most people have great difficulty in knowing just what the right food is. When I ask the mothers of new patients what they consider a good breakfast, snack, or proper meal, they almost invariably describe a diet high in refined carbohydrates, such as sugared refined cereals and pizzas. I then demonstrate to them what these "good" breakfasts are doing to their children's blood sugar curves. They are shocked, but they are more open-minded about a better way of nourishing their offspring.

A small pilot study in the Arlington, Texas, school system similarly revealed that not one mother knew what a good breakfast was. The bill of fare at home commonly consisted of the usual cereals (sugar coated), pop tarts, juice, and milk. The cereals had had the husks removed in milling, thereby losing many B-vitamins and other essential nutrients. Essential biologic minerals and trace elements had been removed. Yet these cereals were the "mainstays" of breakfast eaten in one household after another.

It seems no coincidence that both the behavior and the nutrition of our children are deteriorating at the same time. This is because the American family, generally, is eating the diet that causes the malnutrition of affluence. One of the first things the doctor discovers, when he starts restricting the refined carbohydrates in a child's diet, is how commonly accepted these poor eating habits have become. "Why, that's what we all have for supper!" a mother will gasp when she is told that ice cream, pie, jellies, and other desserts will have to go. The caffeinated drinks, such as tea and colas, are put on the forbidden list and the mother realizes that's what her whole family drinks.

To many conscientious parents, the list of prohibited foods hits them straight between the eyes; it is an emotional shock to find out these "fun" foods are the cause of serious disorders.

Another mother may remonstrate, "It's going to be hard to get him off of ice cream, because his daddy likes ice cream."

In many families this undoubtedly will be a problem. Ideally, the entire family should go on a similar program, for all would benefit. Certainly, cutting out sugary desserts would be good for anyone. But if the ideal situation can't be arranged, then steps must be taken to treat the afflicted child differently, so he will not consume the risky foods that affect his behavior. The cooperation of both parents is essential. If the father allows the child to eat, as a "reward" or "treat," from the forbidden list, the child will not recover. By the same token, if the entire family takes a considerate attitude and sharply curtails its own intake of refined carbohydrates, the child will profit by the example. On the other hand, the child will not be helped by having to watch siblings or parents wolf down the same sweet foods or caffeinated drinks that he can't have. If such foods must be eaten, they should be consumed away from the child.

The Abuse of Television

For its contribution to children's poor eating habits, television has come under serious attack. At the heart of the controversy is an economic concept that is relatively new to modern merchandising: direct selling to children via TV ads. Joan Gussow, a nutrition writer who testified before a Senate subcommittee in 1972, spelled out some of the objectional aspects of television promotion of food products to children. She and others monitored 388 network commercials during a week of viewing children's TV programs and learned that 82 percent of the commercials involved food, drink, and vitamin pill ads directed at children.

Considerably more than the surface message was involved, Gussow testified. Eating behavior is taught. Repeatedly, the ads make sweet appeals. They urge children to eat the worst type of food and swallow the worst type of drinks. Children are being lured into wanting the worst cereals that man has designed. Anything that is "fun, sweet, sparkly, gay, colorful, thick and chocolately, magicky, or crunchily delicious" will eventually parade before the youngsters' eyes on the living room screen. Even vitamins become a vehicle for implanting the belief that if a child doesn't eat right it won't much matter—if he takes his vitamins. The major thrust, with the unstated thesis that only sweetened products are good, leaves a total impact, Gussow reported, that is "blatantly anti-nutrition."

Two equally vocal critics appearing before the Senate Select Committee on Nutrition and Human Needs in 1973—Peggy Charren and Evelyn Sarson, officers of the nonprofit Action for Childrens Television—reported their study in the Boston area: One channel unleashed 67 commercial messages, urging children to eat or drink sweetly-flavored products, during seven hours of a Saturday. This amounted to nearly ten times an hour.

"Were children to eat as much candy and sweetened snacks as the television suggests," they said, "they would never have the appetite for anything else. Adults whom the children respect—father-figures, famous athletes, competent older children—are hourly heard encouraging children to eat candy bars, drink soft drinks, and make friends by sharing snacks. The familiar cartoon characters, the friendly announcer, the superstars all entice children to try the latest sweet snack.

Cereal, one of the hallowed basics, a food children are taught to eat as part of a balanced diet, has become saturated with sugar and is advertised, in many cases, only on the questionable merit of being super sweet. Dr. Jean Mayer, professor of nutrition at Harvard University, warns that many of the children's sweetened cereals are 50 percent sugar—as much as some candy bars.

Charren and Sarson also brought up a number of other disturbing aspects of this sweet pitch directed at minor children. It "sets up a conflict between the parent and child and, in fact, between the child and any number of authority figures—doctors, dentists, and teachers as well as parents." It also shatters the traditional legal protection that children have had. As minors, children are sheltered from entering into sales agreements and other business contracts, wherein their inexperience may be exploited. Federal laws regulate their employment. Yet, as consumers they now are the targets of a bombardment of hard sells, unsurpassed by anything an adult has to face.

"In the world of television," testified Charren and Sarson, "a child is treated as an adult from the day he begins watching television. We recognize in real life that our children are not sophisticated enough to plan the family's meals, and yet on television we expect them to show the most amazing degree of sophistication in coping with the barrage of demands from the most persuasive selling medium of all."

They concluded on a warning note that unless the trend is changed, "we can expect a continued growth of heart disease, hypertension, and poor dental health—the diseases that result from poor eating habits established in childhood which cripple and kill in adulthood."

It is a small wonder that millions of our children suffer continuously from sugar abuse, especially the concentrated carbohydrates found in their super-sweet daily diets. This inundation of sugar leads to a breakdown of regulatory mechanisms in their metabolism. What is even more disturbing is the indication in research done with both humans and rats showing that, once poor diets are established, they may persist. Protein-starved rats normally prefer protein over sugar; but in one experiment researchers P. T. Young and J. P. Chaplin reported that a sugar preference established before the starvation period persisted even when the needs for protein grew. The implications of this are a useful warning; even when protein levels are seemingly adequate, a child may still become hooked on sugar. It is probably that in some children the effects of this sugar abuse may be masked for a period of time, only to erupt as symptoms at a later date. The absence of obvious clinical signs of a disorder does not necessarily mean that all is well. Disease develops slowly, sometimes over decades. The best plan is to *prevent* the end results of sugar and refined starch abuse before they appear, by curtailing these refined substances in the diet.

I have found in my own clinic that, as important as protein is, it is not enough when the individual abuses sugar. Almost invariably, a sugary or high-starch diet means that beneficial nutrients have been omitted from the menu. A perfect illustration of this is Morris, aged four. One of Morris' chief complaints was insomnia; he would get up at night and would be found eating. His speech was confused, and he suffered from a wide range of disorders and misbehavior: running away in all kinds of weather; frequent diarrhea; inattention and tantrums; ceaseless activity; kicking adults in the shins; frequent colds; and headaches.

A diet history (with the suspicious foods italicized) provided immediate clues to Morris' problems:

BREAKFAST

Peanuts
Sausage or ham
Juice

MORNING SNACK

Fritos and *bean dip* (*sugar added*)
Coca-Cola or juice

LUNCH

Peanut butter (*sugar added*)
Cheese
Fritos
Bread (not whole grain)

AFTERNOON SNACK

Fruit
Honey

DINNER

Meat
Noodles and *white crackers*
Milk
Ice cream or *pudding*

BEDTIME

Juice

As I analyzed Morris' diet, I found that he had an adequate supply of protein, but he was deficient in the three other food groups. He definitely was suffering from sugar abuse and consuming far more calories than he needed. Unadulterated peanut butter is good food, but Morris was eating a brand that was hydrogenated, and both the peanut butter and the bean dip had sugar added. Through a computer analysis of his diet, I was able to show Morris' mother that he was receiving the equivalent of *81* teaspoons of sugar a day, by combining estimates of the actual sugar with the equivalent produced from refined carbohydrates such as noodles, crackers, corn chips, pudding, ice cream, and honey. (See Appendix C as a guide to the "hidden" sugars contained in various foods.) But because the overdose of sugar and refined starch crowded out beneficial nutrition, he was deficient in grains and cereals, vegetables and fruit, and dairy products. He was eating 2400 calories a day, 800 more than his recommended daily allowance of 1600, and his actual intake of total carbohydrates, 290 grams, far exceeded the recommended 60 grams.*

---

*See Figure 1.5, page 000, for daily carbohydrates requirements and Figure 2.1, page 000, for caloric recommendations. Using these charts and the Carbohydrate Gram Counter you may devise a chart of your own for monitoring your child's nutrition and establishing general guidelines for health.

When his mother eliminated the suspect items and added wholesome ones, Morris began to improve immediately. In his case the protein intake was adequate and thus did not have to be increased. Most of all, his case illustrated that sugar abuse can overwhelm the good that protein may do and that a complete, balanced meal is necessary for health. Another youngster might exist on Morris' diet without such a gamut of symptoms, but this would not mean that child was escaping the ravages of inferior nutrition. Despite our biochemical differences, the diet that does harm to one person cannot be expected to help another.

Now let's turn to an extreme example of how sugar abuse may affect a psychotic mind. Harold, a teen ager, had come to me with a lifetime of dietary abuse behind him. Very obese, he was depressed, hyperactive, easily fatigued, and at times tearful. He would never finish his school work and had dropped out of school at fifteen. He slept twelve hours a day—from 2 A.M. until 2 P.M. He was clumsy and accident prone. Some of his actions were bizarre: building gun silencers and caskets, chopping off the heads of baby birds, slitting a cat's throat. His parents were desperate.

What was he eating? A lot of everything, especially sugar and refined starch. His "breakfast" was a quart of cola—nothing else. The rest of the day, futilely trying to keep up his blood sugar and energy level, he drank soda and ate pie and cake, along with whatever else he had. Over the duration of a day he would drink a pint of whiskey. His bedtime "snack" was four or five hamburgers, washed down by a quart of cola. Despite his daily consumption of what I figured came to 7,600 calories, he was perpetually hungry. The reason for this was that his system was so swamped with sugar and starches that he

70

never enjoyed a steady, normal blood sugar level. His energy was sapped by "quick energy" items.

The tragedy of Harold's case is that he dropped out of the nutritional program before it had a chance to work. Undoubtedly, he also would have benefitted from psychological counseling, but by then he was in such a far-advanced stage of affluent malnutrition that improvement appeared hopeless unless some new motivating factor entered his life. We can speculate, though, that Harold's tragedy could have been prevented, by modifying his disastrous nutritional regime much earlier in his life. The sooner a poor diet is corrected, the less damage is suffered by the brain and other organs of the body, and the sooner the child may recover from his poorly nourished state.

As I have said before, our pets often have a far better chance of getting a balanced, nutritious diet than do our children. Given the same highly-refined carbohydrate foods that our children eat, our pets would fall sick, become nervous or listless, and in time perish. The human does not age as fast as a dog or a cat, or we might see more casualties among our children than we do.

Nutrition of our pets is not taken for granted. When it comes to pets, the commercial theme is one of protection and health, instead of exploitation. I found striking evidence of this when I recently studied the ingredients of a popular puppy formula. The chow was designed to take care of the dog's energy and growth needs during his first year of life, a period roughly comparable to the human child's development to early adult life. Among other nutrients, the formula contained bone meal, dried milk and whey, wheat germ meal, brewers yeast, vitamins A, D, B_{12}, E, K, B_6, choline, biotin, folic acid, niacin, pantothenic acid, iron, and the trace elements manganese, zinc, copper, and cobalt. (A dog, unlike a human being, synthesizes its own vitamin C and does not require supplementation or intake from food.) It comes as a shock to realize that we often do not give as much thought to the needs of our growing children, our next generation.

Symptoms and Danger Signals

Over many years of practicing pediatrics, I have detected a pattern of the malnutrition of affluence that includes symptoms (subjective evidence, discernible to the patient but not to the doctor), signs (objective evidence that the doctor and others can see), and laboratory findings. These three lists may be of help to you in assessing whether your child is suffering to some degree from this late twentieth-century deficiency disease. Of course, these symptoms sometimes will reflect other disorders, as well.

SYMPTOMS

1. Hunger, snacking, and excessive eating.
2. In some, poor appetite.
3. Headaches.
4. Fatigue, shortness of breath, lack of stamina and muscle tone, lack of strength.
5. Lack of interest and enthusiasm.
6. Nervousness, hyperactivity, and short attention span.
7. Inability to get along with other children.
8. Failing or declining grades.
9. Vague, isolated, and diverse pains.
10. Dizziness and trouble focusing the eyes.
11. Gas and/or constipation.
12. Susceptibility to upper respiratory tract, gastrointestinal, skin, and urinary infections.

13. Up late at night.
14. Hand tremors.
15. Awkward body motions.

SIGNS

1. Postural slump of fatigue.
2. Putty gray pallor.
3. Expressionless face.
4. Dry scaly skin and swollen hair follicles on back of upper arms and anterior thighs.
5. Flushing of periphery of palms, particularly the thumb and little finger edges of the palm.
6. Tenderness above the kidneys if blood sugar drops below 40 milligrams percent.
7. Sullen, suspicious, disinterested manner.
8. Reactive increase in blood pressure of adolescents, thirteen and up, of 180/90.
9. Mild increase in heart rate (90–120) and transiently irregular heart beats.
10. Impulsive anxious speech and movements.
11. Poor physique, either obese or thin and wirey.

LABORATORY FINDINGS
IN MALNUTRITION OF AFFLUENCE

1. Mild anemia.
2. Blood potassium near the lower limits of normal.
3. Variable calcium and phosphorus levels, with abnormal calcium/phosphorus ratios (greater or less than 2 parts calcium to 1 part phosphorus).
4. Blood protein near the lowest limit of the normal range (with normal range 6–8 milligrams percent).
5. Eosinophile cells ("allergy" white cells) in the blood slightly elevated in number.

73

6. Total basophile cell count (a type of white cell) lower than 10 (normal: 10-90).

7. Iron, sodium, potassium, manganese, and chromium often low in hair analysis.

8. Glucose dysglycemia (disturbed blood sugar levels) with glucose tolerance test or food utilization test (test for effects of food and drink on blood sugar).

In the next chapter I will go into greater detail about how the malnutrition of affluence has a major impact upon a key factor in a child's life—his general health.

4

Building Resistance Against Illness

Brenda's case isn't the kind that doctors enjoy talking about. She seemed to be perpetually sick. But although she was receiving very sophisticated medical care, she wasn't getting any better. She soon became a symbol of the frustrations encountered when a sick child is treated without taking her nutrition into consideration.

A bright, attentive four-year-old, she had a sore throat almost constantly. She scarcely had a let-up from repeated colds and bronchitis. She also had severe asthma and high fevers complicated her throat infections. Once Brenda had even been hospitalized for a week as the result of dehydration brought on by vomiting and high fever.

Over and over she returned to the doctor. He treated her vigorously with the best medicines that science had developed: antihistamines to control her sneezing, drainage, and coughing; penicillin and other drugs to combat her throat infections, high fever, and vomiting. For the past two winters she had been taking gamma

75

globulin injections monthly to build up her resistance. Yet Brenda remained sick most of the time, gaining little more than temporary relief. She didn't know what it was to be well.

Accompanied by her tearful mother, Brenda was pale, breathing with the short, rapid, pants that are characteristic of asthma, and seemingly emotionless when she first appeared in my office.

Despite all that had been done for Brenda previously, she had never been given a thorough nutritional evaluation. It was soon apparent where some of her trouble lay when I found out about her diet.

BREAKFAST

Dry cereal with *cinnamon, sugar,* and *raisins*
Orange juice
(Raisins and orange juice are also high in natural sugar, which in the absence of protein will add to the sugar overdose)
An egg twice a week
Milk occasionally

MORNING SNACK

Cola
Sweet roll

LUNCH

Peanut butter and *jelly*
Cake
Sweetened pop
Turkey scraps occasionally

DINNER

Meat or chicken
Some vegetables

Milk
Pie or *cake*

BEDTIME SNACK

Cake or *sweet roll* or *cookies*

It was easy to see from Brenda's diet history that she was suffering from a surfeit of refined carbohydrates, both sugars and starches. To gain a more precise insight into how Brenda's endocrine system was handling the flood of sugar, I administered a five-hour glucose tolerance test. Her fasting blood sugar was very good, but after she had swallowed the test glucose, her blood sugar curve shot up too fast too soon and then steadily declined. At the third hour it went into a nose-dive and remained about 40 milligrams below her fasting level for the remainder of the test. Her resistance to disease and germs was very low.

The diagnosis was confirmed: sugar and refined starch abuse. Even if other causes were involved, the obvious thing to do was to correct this problem first. But in order to have a more in-depth analysis of Brenda's eating habits, I had a computer study made of the data her mother provided. Although her caloric intake of 1500 calories daily was about right for her age, there were many problem areas. She ate 200 grams of carbohydrates and most of her carbohydrate foods were of the refined variety. She should have been eating *half* as much carbohydrate foods, with all of them complex carbohydrates from vegetables, fruits, whole-grain cereals and breads. She was deficient in methionine, an amino acid that is vital to antibody or germ-fighter synthesis, and her calcium intake was strikingly low. The computer study, in this case, was helpful to demonstrate to the parents what exactly happens when a child eats the foods that Brenda did.

Figure 4-1. Brenda's Glucose Tolerance Test

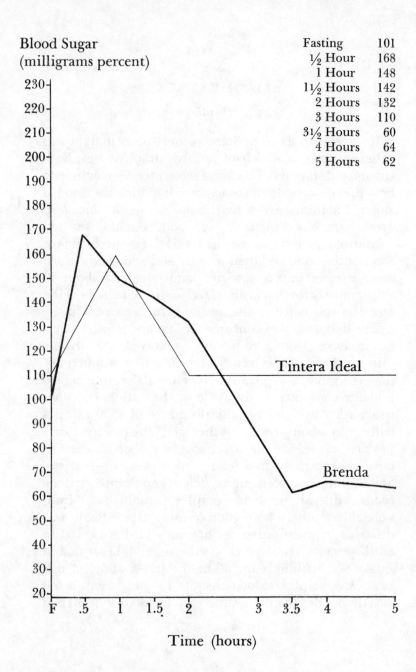

Fasting	101
½ Hour	168
1 Hour	148
1½ Hours	142
2 Hours	132
3 Hours	110
3½ Hours	60
4 Hours	64
5 Hours	62

Blood Sugar (milligrams percent)

Tintera Ideal

Brenda

Time (hours)

Brenda was sick when she came in, and some antibiotics had to be prescribed to help alleviate her current symptoms. But the drugs were used in relatively small doses and it was explained that this was but a temporary solution. The real approach to treatment would be to create a state of full health that would help her prevent a repetition of her medical difficulties.

This meant that Brenda must build up her *host resistance*. Resistance is the major key to health at any age. If your child's resistance is high, he is likely to enjoy his health fully and will not catch every "bug" that comes along. His body's defenses will be strong and will rout any would-be invader.

Nothing is more essential to building host resistance than proper nutrition. Most people are unaware that foods can be classified as to whether they build resistance or promote susceptibility to disease and degeneration. Eggs, liver, fresh vegetables and fruit, for instance, are resistance foods, because they provide the body its raw materials and promote health. On the other hand, table sugar, caffeinated and sweetened soda, and white-flour products are susceptibility foods; they weaken the body's resistance and should be eliminated and replaced with resistance foods. This is important for children of all ages, but especially for those whose resistance has been lowered by chronic sickness. Resistance foods arm the child with the factors that help resist infections, colds, and even more serious disorders; they help his blood sugar attain a state of homeostasis, or stability, so that he is more likely to feel well.

Brenda was started on a nutritional regimen that took *all sugar* from her diet. This included a prohibition even on orange juice, because of its easily-absorbed natural sugars. Her Carbohydrate Control Program set her limit for complex starches and other carbohydrates in fruits, vegetables, breads, and cereals at 100 grams a day. And because Brenda needed to be built up, she was placed on a high protein diet that called for, along with her other whole food, six protein feedings per day: an egg for breakfast; beef, mutton, organ cuts, chicken, or fish at lunch and dinner; and small snack servings of cheese, unsweetened yogurt, or meat between meals and before going to bed. These were *resistance foods*. Protein helps stabilize the blood sugar at an even level and builds antibodies or germ fighters. In her case, supplements were also needed, to provide her with the B-complex, C, and general vitamins, plus tablets for calcium and magnesium.

Brenda did not get well overnight. But she showed noticeable improvement as the weeks went by, and the office visits tapered down remarkably. Gradually, she became free of the high temperatures that had dogged her. Antibiotics were becoming a thing of the past, because her body, with a grand assist from nutritional therapy, was doing the splendid job it had been designed to do.

The Chronically Sick Child

One of the most consistently ignored problems in modern medicine is that of the chronically sick child who has no serious organic disease. A child like Brenda is not seriously ill; she is just sick all the time with minor ailments. Such a condition should not be ignored, with the hope the child will outgrow it. Any child who is sick as often as Brenda was in the early years of life is setting a pattern of ill health that makes her a candidate for a serious illness which may some day materialize.

Brenda's case gives us a hint of the overall health problems facing children in this country. Most pediatricians are harried beyond endurance, especially during the winter, as they repeatedly treat colds in the same children, with the monotony broken only by complaints of abscessed ears, tonsillitis, bronchitis, asthma, runny noses, and devastating bouts with diarrhea and vomiting.

Many children are overweight, although this was not the condition that brought them to the doctor. The older obese child is one of the greatest challenges in pediatrics, for the extremely fat child almost always presents a psychological as well as a physical problem. The best opportunity for success in treating obesity is with the grade school child or younger, simply because it is easier to control his environment and, therefore, diet.

The drug bills for some families with chronically sick children run as high as $80 to $100 a month. Yet the conventional approach to colds is usually limited to the prescription of antihistamines and antibiotics. These drugs are not always effective, however, and researchers have now learned that antihistamines can gum up secretions so that they stick in the ears and bronchial tubes and cling to hoarse vocal cords. Even the simple application of common aspirin in large doses may present a risk, especially to small children, inducing internal bleeding and poisoning. After all, like other drugs, aspirin is a substance foreign to the human body.

Whichever weapon is chosen in the conventional drug attack on these common illnesses, the plight of the child is not a happy one.

The first stage of treatment, of course, must be to rule out the possibility of any organic disease, if the child has suffered chronically for a long period of time. This is true whether or not he is being treated by a nutritional-oriented pediatrician. He may need a chest X-ray, if chronic asthma is suspected. If the child does not listen to others, he could be partially deaf from accumulation of cold mucous behind his eardrums. Severe stomach

81

complaints may require a gastrointestinal series of X-rays. All intense headaches are not migraine or allergy-caused, and all neurological disturbances are not due to low blood sugar.

For example, one child was brought to me complaining of severe headaches. The mother believed these pains were caused by low blood sugar, but careful questioning and a thorough physical examination revealed the headaches to be a result of a massive brain tumor. Indeed, the brain surgeon stated that the tumor was the largest of its type he had ever removed from a child of that age.

Once an organic disease has been ruled out, however, careful attention should be given to the chronic condition. Continuing affliction with "common" disorders like runny noses and colds and "minor" infections can become very serious. Most of all, it could be an harbinger of an unhappy, unhealthy future. Drs. Emanuel Cheraskin and W. Marshall Ringsdorf, Jr., have concluded that, "in reality, most chronic diseases are pediatric in origin." It is in childhood that the basis is laid for serious and chronic diseases of later life: cardiovascular diseases, diabetes, even cancer. Most chronic conditions are extremely slow in developing.

Cheraskin and Ringsdorf, citing data from the National Center for Health Statistics, have shown that there has been a dramatic increase in chronic conditions in the seventeen-to-twenty-four-year-old age group. In 1962, a total of 37.7 percent of these young people had one or more chronic conditions; by 1967, the percentage was 44.6—an increase of almost 7 percent in five years!

These are young people who should be in the best of health. Obviously something must have happened to them in their early years. Chronic conditions do not occur overnight.

The contributions of Dr. Hans Selye, the distinguished

director of the Institute of Experimental Medicine and Surgery at the University of Montreal, give us some insight into how serious these chronic illnesses may be, "minor" or otherwise. Dr. Selye discovered the General Adaptation Syndrome, the body's nonspecific reaction to all kinds of stress, which he defines as "essentially the *wear and tear* in the body caused by life at any one time." Chronic illness, such as Brenda experienced, is clearly a form of stress that Selye was talking about. He observed that all these symptoms, such as Brenda had, could be summed up as the "syndrome of just being sick." The body has one general means of reacting to any form of wear and tear, resulting in a hormonal reaction from the adrenals. The more prolonged the stress, whether the stress of sickness, of sugar abuse, or of other source, the greater the damage, ultimately exhausting the ability of the adrenals and other organs to respond appropriately.

Perhaps this concept of a basic disorder in all sickness at least partially explains why so many children today are unable to ingest sugar—or metabolize even good, natural fruit sugars as are in fruit and fruit juices—without their blood sugar going up, far above normal, and then down, far below normal. A normal child should be able to ingest the glucose test load without these abnormal patterns. It leaves us wondering what, in their brief lives, their eating habits have done to so radically disrupt their bodies' functions.

It is well to remember that, unless these "minor" problems are corrected or prevented, the chronic colds and runny noses of childhood may be laying the groundwork for a serious health crisis in adult life. The time to do something, of course, is now, whatever the present age of the child or youth. Whatever the child's medical history, something can be done to improve his health through nutrition. Improving his nutrition will support whatever treatment the doctor is providing.

Most of all, if your child appears to be healthy now, or at least has no symptoms, this is the time to improve his nutrition, in order to *prevent* nutritionally-linked health problems later on.

Nutrition During Pregnancy

A child's nutritional needs change with his age and weight. In most instances, these changes amount to increased energy needs (more calories)—a matter of quantity rather than the type of food. However, there are several stages of a child's growth that do have some distinguishing differences other than those of overall food intake. In order to analyze your child's nutritional requirements systematically, it will help to take a look at the stages of growth from prenatal life through puberty.

The most important time of life for the child, nutritionally, is before birth. The best time to get the child off to a healthy start is during his prenatal life, through the mother's providing sound nutrition for herself during pregnancy. The developing fetus gains every milligram of nourishment from its mother during these nine months, as she passes all the required nutrients via the umbilical cord to the baby. For this reason, a mother-to-be should begin thinking about her child's nutrition even before conception. In order to make conditions ideal for the conception and subsequent fetal life of an infant, both parents should be in good health and well nourished.

After conception, the mother especially should pay close attention to what she eats, making sure she has a balanced diet that is generous in vitamins, minerals, and especially protein. What the mother eats will provide the raw material from which a new human being will be created. We might think of the fertilized ovum as the blueprint. This blueprint is not enough for building a new life; the mother herself must supply the construction materials, which come from her body, primarily from the food she ingests.

Dr. Roger J. Williams has shown that nutrition, especially during the prenatal months, is crucial to the proper development of a baby. While we can assume that a sick mother may produce a sick baby, the fact that the mother may feel reasonably well, despite a poor diet, does not mean the developing baby may not suffer. Additionally, it is well to realize that, as Dr. Williams reports, "no part of the body is exempt from poor development if the individual has been supplied with deficient nutrition." The degree of damage may range from very mild to exceedingly severe, and the brain is likely to be an organ affected if any of the essential nutrients are not adequately supplied. As Dr. Williams points out in *Nutrition Against Disease*, what is important is that a specific deficiency does not mean that harm is limited to a particular part of the body that needs that nutrient. Every part of the body needs the essential food elements. Calcium is needed for more than development of teeth and bones, iron is required for more than healthy blood.

Dr. Williams recommends 50 milligrams of pantothenic acid, a B vitamin that he discovered, to every mother-to-be; it helps prevent reproductive failure and aids in withstanding stress. Just as pantothenic acid is needed all over the body, the same is generally true of the other essential vitamins and minerals. For instance, vitamin B_6 (pyridoxine) is extremely important in the nutrition of a pregnant woman; Dr. John M. Ellis, a leading clinical authority on vitamin B_6, has reported 50 to 100 milligrams or more daily is useful in preventing the edema (swelling/water retention) of pregnancy. The scientific literature has demonstrated that B_6 deficiency can be a factor in birth defects. The point is that *all* of the essential nutrients are needed, and are necessary for the developing baby as well as the mother.

It is important to remember that the fetus does not necessarily "rob" the mother for what it needs, if her nutrition is inadequate. In some instances the fetus may get some of its requirements in this way, but in order to err on the side of safety it is well to remember that zinc, one of our trace minerals, can come only from food or supplements. Experiments with rats have shown that zinc from the mother's skeleton is not shared with the developing rat fetus. This means, as Dr. Williams has emphasized, that "when there is a zinc deficiency in the diet during pregnancy, the mother may not suffer from the deficiency, but the offspring will."

While this may not be the case for every other element used to build the newly-forming body, it is a wise pregnant woman who will act as if the same fact held true for all of the nutritional factors. Then she will enjoy a diet containing everything both she and her baby need.

Certainly a woman should make an appointment with her obstetrician at the first suspicion that she may be pregnant, so that she can be advised on supplements and diet, as well as get a general checkup at the outset. In addition, researchers have also issued warnings about smoking cigarettes at any time during pregnancy and about taking drugs, which include not only addictive "street" drugs but also alcohol. Even moderate drinking by the mother-to-be is now recognized as a risk that, with other factors, may result in a premature birth, low birth weight of the infant, or growth problems. Some studies have implicated alcohol in facial deformities of the baby.

The First Year of Life

The next most important time of the baby's life, nutritionally speaking, is immediately following birth. The first "growth spurt" comes during early infancy, until around the child's first birthday.

In infancy, as during the prenatal period, the baby should receive its nourishment from the mother, through breast feeding. Although the trend in this country for decades has been to bottle feed, the scientific evidence remains in favor of the breast-fed baby. Happily, there are indications of a growing percentage of breast-feeding mothers in recent years.

At the Ninth International Congress of Nutrition, held in Mexico City in 1972, the consensus was that a baby should be breast-fed for the first six months, at least. Authorities such as Drs. Paul György and D. B. Jeliffe called attention to the fact that bottle feeding may lead to obesity in later years, as well as a lowered resistance to certain bacteria. The reason for this is that the bottle formula usually contains more calories than the baby needs, as most "formulas" are laced with unneeded sugar. Thus the pattern is set for more fat cells in later life. Furthermore, mother's milk—the human species' own natural food for its young, developed for its especial needs over the hundreds of thousands of years—contains antibodies that protect the infant from a wide range of bacteria. Cow's milk or soybean substitute formulas do not provide these natural defenses.

Bottle feeding, Dr. György asserted, is a symptom of an affluent society; in the United States, the infant is commonly given a bottle supplement in the hospital during the first five days of life. Put another way, we could say that the malnutrition of affluence begins in the cradle, if not in the womb.

Although Dr. Jane Pitt, professor of pediatrics at Columbia Presbyterian Medical Center, as recently as 1977, reported studies proving that breast-fed babies had significantly fewer illnesses than bottle-fed babies, the evidence has been available for decades that breast feeding is a superior way of infant nutrition. A Chicago study in 1929, involving 383 children whose ages ranged from seven to thirteen, concluded that those who had been breast-fed were, on the whole, both physically and mentally superior to the bottle-fed. Children who had been breast-fed from periods ranging from four to nine months were assessed as being superior in all ways to all other groups and had the highest percentage of bright children. On the other hand, those in the bottle-fed group were more susceptible to disease and were the slowest to learn to talk and to walk.

As the principal food during this period of rapid development, milk especially contributes calcium that promotes bone growth. Each species takes care of its young through the mother's milk; this means that human milk is ideal for the human infant. There are significant differences between breast milk and cow's milk. Breast milk is higher in whey than is cow's milk, while cow's milk is higher in its principal protein, casein. Casein makes such a big curd that the baby has difficulty getting it out of his stomach. Babies have immature kidneys, which can't properly handle the end product of the metabolism of excess protein. Breast milk is higher in oleic fatty acid and lower in linoleic acid, and this is what enhances the absorption of calcium from breast milk. Cow's milk is too high in phosphorus for humans, and the high phosphorus content will depress the calcium blood levels. For these reasons, great care must be taken with infant feeding. Too many mothers give their babies too much phosphorus. By breast feeding, however, these risks are taken care of automatically.

The only problems that may be encountered with mother's milk are its variable quality and the transmission of any toxic and harmful substances that the mother may have ingested. There is rarely a problem of quantity in a rested, well-nourished mother, as long as the baby is allowed to nurse regularly and as long as he wishes. Nor is there a problem of the baby's becoming allergic to his mother's milk. In some instances the mother may transmit her own allergic antibodies through the milk, but these are to what *she* may be allergic, not to what the baby may be allergic. For example, if the mother is allergic to cow's milk or another food and produces antibodies to it, and the mother drinks cow's milk while nursing, the baby will have a reaction to the cow's milk as a result of the mother's antibodies. He will not be reacting to his mother's breast milk. This is known as *passive* response of the infant to breast milk, and his own active immune response is *not* involved. This is much less of a problem than a baby's allergic reaction to cow's milk "formula," which is a frequent and serious medical complication in the newborn.

However, the fact that the mother can transmit certain substances through the milk is a further reason why she should insure that her own diet be as solid as it was during pregnancy. She should not eat junk foods, caffein, nor should she smoke or drink alcohol. A good way to tell if your doctor is nutritionally minded is to see if he takes a good diet history of the lactating mother. The pediatrician should compile a diet history for the mother as well as for the child.

For new mothers who may not enjoy sufficient self-confidence in breast-feeding, there exists in most communities a local chapter of La Leche League, an organization of mothers devoted to the natural and most practical way of nursing their babies. These mothers may provide helpful information as well as emotional support when there is a nursing problem.

In the cases where nonhuman milk is fed the baby, care should be taken *not* to add sugar or syrup to the formula. By avoiding unnecessary sugar at this age, the mother may be preventing a host of nutritional and physiological problems for the child at a later stage. The caloric needs can be met with appropriate complex carbohydarates.

Vitamin drops also may be introduced in infancy, to provide vitamins C and D. The recommended daily allowance for vitamin C is 35 milligrams for the child from birth to age one year, while 400 international units of vitamin D is required. As we saw earlier, the child can synthesize vitamin D from sunshine if there is adequate exposure to the sun, but certainly during the winter months when there are fewer opportunities for this, vitamin D drops or cod liver oil may be needed. The emphasis, whether in exposure to the sun or vitamin D supplementation, should be on a *sufficiency*, while avoiding a surplus—a sunburn is no fun and is not healthy. Vitamin drops that contain recommended daily allowances of vitamins A, C, D, and the B-complex may especially be helpful for babies who are not breast fed.

The best time to instutute proper feeding habits is in infancy. Although breast-feeding is recommended for at least six months, the introduction of solid foods may begin at around three months of age. This is the ideal age for the child to take his first step toward a well-directed adult life by learning how to handle a new food. Food at this age should be given in very small amounts to avoid laying the groundwork for obesity in the future.

The following technique has never failed in my practice of pediatrics:

1. First, give the baby 2 ounces of breast milk or formula to keep him from being hungry. (If breast feeding, the milk can be hand-expressed with a breast pump.)

2. Use ½ to 1 teaspoonful of strained, noncommercial meat thinned with formula milk or breast milk. Such a small amount of meat can be prepared at home with little difficulty, thereby avoiding any undesired additives or sugar in the commercial varieties.

3. Take one-third of a teaspoonful of the milk-meat mixture and put it under the infant's upper gums, and follow it with milk.

4. Repeat the process until all of the strained meat is used.

The point, in the beginning, is to insure that the baby becomes acquainted with new, solid food while milk is still the major source of nutrition and energy. There is no pressure for the baby to be weaned from the breast or bottle. The baby can play with his solid food, push it from his mouth, roll it around, or blow it out. He is getting familiarized with the new food, and the parent is working toward the eventual goal in which the child is both well fed and well trained.

Introducing the strained meat at this stage is very important. Once the baby has accepted meat, as he will if the parent exhibits patience, then the highest hurdle has been passed. Strained vegetables are then much easier to introduce. This small quantity—one-half or one teaspoon of meat three times a day—is just enough for him to taste and learn to like. Solid food at this age is not yet essential to his metabolism, so it doesn't matter if it takes six days or several months for him to get used to the new food. If he gags or sputters at first, let him. A relaxed approach is always helpful. Don't give up, and don't be afraid of your baby!

While avoiding all commercial baby foods and juices because of additives and concentrated carbohydrates, you may later gradually add "bonus" foods to the growing baby's diet. By the time he is weaned he should be handling cottage cheese, yogurt, buttermilk, and strained fish as well as strained meats and vegetables. Eggs shouldn't be offered during the first six months because of the possibilities of allergy at that early stage. By the age of one year, the child should be able to eat all foods in a strained version. Most health food stores have baby food grinders that sell for a small sum, which will solve the preparation problem.

The Preschool Years

For the next several years, from ages one to around five or six, the child needs very little food for healthy development. Following this period of "explosive growth in the first year of life, he reaches a "plateau" stage and growth is more gradual and almost unnoticed. *What* he eats is far more important than *how much* he eats. This especially applies to milk during preschool years. At this age the child needs only 16 ounces or two glasses of milk a day for perfect growth. Furthermore, cheese and eggs, in relatively small daily amounts, can be used as *complete substitutes* for milk.

It is not until the age of two and a half to three years that the child can usually handle any type of unstrained food. The reason for this is that he does not have enough teeth to adequately chew with side-to-side motions. If the more solid foods aren't properly chewed, then they will go through the intestines whole and undigested.

The one-to-six age is the danger zone when, as we have seen, children often develop poor eating habits. Ironically, it is the "tons" or "scads" of milk drunk by these children that help destroy what little appetite they should normally have. Large quantities of liquid of any kind—but particularly milk and pop—fill up the stomach and leave no room for essential protein foods.

Children who are living on milk alone will continue to refuse other valuable foods as long as milk is available even in small amounts. For this reason, the first step in correcting protein deficiency and carbohydrate overload of this type is to temporarily eliminate milk *completely* from the child's diet. As startling as this may seem to some parents, children can remain in excellent health, with fine teeth, while drinking no milk over long periods; on the other hand, despite their consuming a great deal of milk, protein-deficient, carbohydrate-swamped children all have poor teeth.

Once the child is solidly on his new nutritional path, milk can be returned to the diet, in the supporting role where it belongs. The appetite-killing sugary and starchy snacks should never again be allowed.

When parents accept that it is all right to let a child go without food until he is hungry, feeding problems will begin to disappear. As long as the child is allowed to choose only from high quality food, particularly protein, and is not offered sugary snacks or refined starches, his normal hunger will propel him toward sensible eating habits.

It is well to remember that during the "plateau" stages of growth the child does not need as much food as he does during the "growth spurt" periods. The fact that a child is burning up energy by running and playing does not mean he requires a huge number of calories. Activity plays a minor part in food requirements at this age.

Early School Years

Realistically speaking, the ages from five to puberty constitute a period of increased growth but not what could be called a "growth spurt." There are really only two growth spurts—during the first twelve months of life and during adolescence. Since the onset of puberty varies from one child to another, there is no precise way to pin down, on the basis of age alone, the limits of the early school years. During these so-called "middle years" when the child has started going to school but has not yet reached adolescence, growth continues but it is slow.

There are no special nutritional needs from age five or six until puberty. There is a gradual increase in various nutrients which can be satisfied by the same foods he ate before starting school, perhaps in slightly larger quantities. The charts in Chapters I and II, pages 000 and 000 give some idea of the increases. As you can see in the case of calcium, there is a progressive need for nutrients from Day One until the end of growth around the ages of eighteen to twenty-two.

The simple truth is that the child should eat properly— a little of all the food groups at *all* ages—with an automatic increase in consumption due to the greater appetite of all boys and girls that reaches its peak at puberty.

I have always prepared my patients' families for this later increased intake and need in my nutritional instructions from early childhood. In the slow growth period from one year to ten years-plus, the parents try to force food down the child when the truth is that he can get along well with one *good* meal a day. I alleviate the worry over picky eating in these years by telling the family, "Wait'll he's a teen ager—you'll have to back a food truck up to the door!" The parents' concern should be with the quality and variety of food, not its quantity.

Puberty and Adolescence

The second great growth spurt in the human occurs during the onset of puberty and adolescence. This is signaled by the appearance of secondary sex characteristics, such as the appearance of pubic hair, the growth of the breasts in the female, and the development of the sexual organs in both male and female. The male's voice tends to deepen. The female begins to menstruate. The sex hormones are activated—testosterone and the gonadotropic hormones in the male, estrogen and progesterone in the female.

There is no precise date for the onset of adolescence. The "endocrine time clock" goes off anywhere from nine to sixteen years in females and twelve to seventeen in males, depending on the individual. However, generally speaking, we can note this major growth spurt as occurring from the ages of nine to eighteen in the female and from ten to twenty-two in the male. By the ages of eighteen in the female and twenty-two in the male, the rapid growth period will have ended. Each child's growth pattern is his own and the best sign of his increased need for nutrients and calories is likely to be his own appetite.

The highest nutrient needs are experienced during this period, which may be labeled either puberty, adolescence, or major growth spurt. It is interesting that the need for some nutrients, such as vitamins A, E, C, B_1, and B_6, increases during this time of adolescence and remains at this level throughout life. However, the requirements for vitamin D remain the same from birth to death, and the need for vitamin B_{12} is the same for both males and females.

The need for calories, though, is higher for males during this period of rapid body growth than for females. Vitamin B-complex requirements, particularly for vitamin B_1, appear to be higher for males throughout life beginning in these years.

During this stage larger amounts of all the known nutrients are required, which means that the adolescent should increase his intake of various foods. Calcium is needed more now for bone growth. Iron needs continue to be higher in the female from puberty until menopause because of monthly blood losses through menstruation. Dietary iron is availalbe in all red meats. The special nutritional needs for males are merely a matter of quantity. They need more of everything because of their increased body mass and metabolic rate.

Adolescent nutritional needs should take care of themselves if the child is fed properly. Assuming that he is getting the right kind of food, his appetite (which is keyed to his growing needs) will work like a thermostat for quantity. It is only the child who was allowed to eat and drink junk food early in life who won't eat right and get enough to eat in the teen years. Unfortunately, some children do not learn to train themselves early and parental permissiveness encourages their behavior. The nutritional deficiencies of adolescence begin with the two-month-old infant who refuses his strained "practice" meat.

If the adolescent consumes the foods I have described in Chapter II, such as dairy products, truits, vegetables, meats whole grain breads, and cereals, and avoids items like sweets, refined starches, and caffein of all sorts, which I have noted in Chapter III, he is not likely to have any problem in filling his needs for growth during this particular time of life.

Malnourishment, Illness, and Stress

If you have been following the guidelines for offering resistance foods and avoiding susceptibility foods, your child is likely to be enjoying better than average health. But what if you are just now getting into a nutritional program and your child's health record has been less than desirable? How can we better understand the links between illness and poor nourishment?

First, malnutrition is a major cause of illness, and illness worsens the state of malnutrition. A severe illness depletes the body, destroying as much as 135 grams of protein in a single day. Infections tax the body's vitamins A and C; gastrointestinal disorders may hamper the synthesis of certain B vitamins. When drugs are used to combat infections, favorable bacteria are killed in the intestines and the process may interfere with the absorption of amino acids.

In research conducted by Dr. Anthony J. Sbarra and associates in Boston, phagocytic effectiveness was shown to be reduced in children suffering from protein-calories malnutrition. The phagocytes (specialized leukocytes or "white cells") in the blood perform two essential functions: they ingest bacteria and, as scavengers, ingest dead tissue and degenerated cells. In other words, healthy phagocytes are not only useful, they are crucial to our resistance to disease. The phagocytes in these children's blood apparently did not engulf or kill bacteria as well as they should have. When the protein-deficient children were placed on a high protein diet with sufficient calories, supplemented with vitamins and iron, their phagocytic action returned to normal. Dr. Sbarra also pointed out that patients with deficiencies in vitamins A and B have an increased susceptibility to infection.

But the most damning proof of all against a common item ingested by today's children came out of an experiment cited by Dr. Emanuel Cheraskin of the University of Alabama Medical Center in Birmingham. It was demonstrated that an individual's capacity to resist infection can be dangerously weakened in as little as forty-five minutes *by dietary means alone.*

Using a sweetened cola, the experiment proved that *the phagocytic index is reduced by 30 percent within 45 minutes of drinking the cola.* The phagocytic index refers to the number of bacteria ingested and destroyed by the phagocytes. As Cheraskin points out, the healthier the phagocyte, the more bacterial bodies it will pick up. Cheraskin then commented that some people can even reduce their phagocytic index by 90 percent in forty-five minutes merely by eating a couple of servings of pie a la mode.

A more elaborate experiment by Dr. Albert Sanchez and associates at Loma Linda University tested the impact of carbohydrates upon the phagocytic index of human volunteers. Six forms of carbohydrate were tested on each volunteer, on six different days. After an overnight fast of about twelve hours, each volunteer was given 100 grams of carbohydrate. The six forms of carbohydrate were: glucose, starch, fructose, sucrose, honey (glucose, 44 percent; fructose, 52 percent; sucrose, 2 percent, dextrin, 2 percent), and orange juice (glucose, 25 percent; fructose, 25 percent). Essentially, then, it was a test of starch and five sugars. Blood was drawn just before ingestion (fasting level) and at intervals up to five hours following ingestion to study the effect upon constituents in the blood.

The results showed that *all* of the sugars (glucose, fructose, sucrose, honey, and orange juice) significantly lowered the phagocytic index. Starch also lowered the index some, but nothing like the sugars. The researchers agreed that there was a significant difference between the effects of the sugars and that of starch, which is a more complex carbohydrate. The mechanism by which the phagocytic index was lowered was through impairment of the leukocytes' function rather than through a decrease in their number. The sugars simply partially disabled the phagocytes' ability to engulf bacteria. The greatest effect was during the first two hours, but it lasted for at least five hours.

The diet that significantly affected the phagocytes in the bloodstreams of the volunteers in these experiments is repeating the performance, often more dramatically, in the systems of our children in every town and city of this country. It is worth noting that similar loads of honey and orange juice produced approximately the same effects as glucose, fructose, and sucrose. The sugars in fruit juices, gram for gram, are similar to those found in purer form. The results of the experiments serve as a warning that if juices are used they should be accompanied by solid, preferably protein, food and should be assessed carefully for their effects upon the child.

Nutritional factors can just as easily be a positive force in combatting illness. At the Western Hemisphere Nutrition Congress V, in Quebec in August, 1977, it was shown that motility—the power of spontaneous movement —of phagocytes is enhanced by protein in the diet.

Added to the sugar effects upon the phagocytic index is the fact that many sugared drinks, especially all colas such as *Coca-Cola* and *Pepsi*, also contain caffein. Beverages that are not always recognized as containing caffein include *Dr. Pepper, Tab*, and all diet colas. The caffein raises, then lowers, a child's blood sugar in much the same way as sugar. The mechanism involves drawing stored sugar from the liver, which accounts for the pick-up, then the let-down, as the sugar is dispersed through many very complex metabolic pathways in the body. Many parents do not realize that there is the caffein equivalent of a half-cup of coffee (40–54 milligrams) in every diet cola, whether it be *Diet Dr. Pepper, Diet Pepsi*, or *Tab*. Additionally, there are 20 milligrams per ounce of caffein in pure chocolate, with somewhat less in chocolate milk.

Recent research also indicates that an allergic phenomenon may play a part in some cases of lowered resistance. Dr. William Bryan, an allergist in St. Louis, has developed a test for allergies with which he studies the impact of the allergy–causing substance upon the white blood cells. In certain patients the total white blood cell count is reduced in proportion to the degree of exposure. This suggests that, at least in those sensitive individuals, the resistance mechanisms are impaired.

All of these factors in the malnutrition–illness cycle are part of the larger picture in children's health and may form a significant share of the stress upon a child. Nutritional stress may be as debilitating as emotional stress from school demands or family situations. As Dr. Hans Selye has pointed out, the end results of stress upon the body are about the same, regardless of the cause. Illness itself is a form of stress; it can increase the body's needs for certain nutrients, just as emotional stress can cause the body to lose large amounts of nutrients, such as vitamins, through accelerated excretion rates. When the body is already deficient in these necessary substances, resistance to germs, viruses, and disease becomes proportionately lower in a child. Reserves have become depleted. Vitamin C, for example, is lost in large quantities from the adrenal cortex during periods of high stress. It is reasonable to replace these constituents, but as Selye, the authority on stress, has indicated, it is not a matter of supplying excessive amounts of one nutrient by itself. A well-balanced diet is never more necessary than when your child is sick.

The case of Gene and his mother aptly illustrates the importance of balance and how a parent can get carried away trying to improve her offspring's health. Gene suffered from cerebral palsy and it appeared that he might have to be institutionalized. His mother was a nervous type, willing to move heaven and earth to help her child. First, she poured buckets, it seemed, of carrot juice down him. The poor boy turned yellow as the result of pigmentation caused by carotenemia, an excess of carotene in the blood. I managed to guide her away from this pitfall, whereupon she began pouring large quantities of brewers yeast down him. In this case, my major role, much of the time, was to curtail the mother's zealousness and to persuade her to take a more moderate approach. As it turned out, Gene did not have to be placed in an institution, because he responded to a program of sensorimotor stimulation, backed up by a balanced nutritional regimen.

"Allergies" That Are Not Allergies

I have learned in my own practice that certain disorders which on the surface appear to be allergies can be treated successfully with nutrition—correcting a poor diet and using the principles I have already discussed to improve nutrition. There are some conditions that are "dead ringers" for allergy. I call them the "great masqueraders."

I must emphasize that I am not talking about life-threatening allergic manifestations, which in all instances should be handled by an allergy specialist. In some severe cases, the patient may go into shock if left untreated.

However, there are some "allergies" that standard allergy treatments fail to clear up. These are not specific allergies to environmental allergens such as pollens, fibers, and foods; instead, the child's allergy-like symptoms seem to be related to his lowered resistance to all stresses.

In such situations, the aim of orthomolecular pediatrics

101

is to raise the child's resistance to all forms of stress—heat, cold, anger, viruses, bacteria, and pollutants—through improvement of the defense mechanisms of the body. This is related to the premise of Hans Selye's general adaptation syndrome. Selye elaborated three stages of the syndrome as follows: first, the alarm reaction (response to challenge); second, the stage of resistance; and third, exhaustion, resulting in permanent and irreversible body damage as the result of prolonged, overwhelming challenge of a weakened body. Stress of any kind, from any source, may eventually bring on the third stage if left to continue its ravages upon the body. The therapeutic goal should be to keep the body's defenses strong so that it can handle whatever stress comes, and thereby prevent any serious damage.

Certainly, building up the body nutritionally is one of the most significant ways to deal with the stresses of life. This also may save the parent as much as $200 for allergy testing, plus weekly injections, which may not be necessary. If the symptoms don't clear up at the second review of the case a month or two later, then I send the child to an allergist.

There is no universal agreement as to what an allergy is, but it is associated with an overreaction of some sort—sneezing, asthma, a runny nose, red or itching eyes, rashes, bloating, and diarrhea, along with irritability, sleeplessness, fatigue, and nervousness. The earliest sign of cow's milk allergy in an infant is diarrhea. A change to soybean milk is usually made by the pediatrician. This may solve the problem or it may only help a little. In any case, care should be taken not to add sugar or syrup to the formula, whatever is done.

As previously stated, the best approach to infant nutrition is breast feeding, which is the most reliable insurance against allergy in the child. When breast milk isn't provided, the next best choice is certified raw goat's or cow's milk. This is milk from disease-free herds that has not been pasteurized or homogenized. Homogenization allows the enzyme xanthine oxidase in small fat globules to enter the body and deposit fat in our arteries. The heating process in pasteurization seems to destroy some of the nutritional components in milk, for I have seen children do much better on certified raw milk than their older brothers or sisters had done on pasteurized milk. A problem, however, is that certified raw milk is often difficult to find. Sometimes health food stores carry it or may provide leads to dairymen who sell it. The important thing about certified raw milk is to make certain the equipment used in processing it is clean, and it is worth checking this out personally at the diary.

By controlling the complex carbohydrates and by deleting the unnecessary refined ones, the nonspecific diarrheas of childhood almost always improve. Older children, including those who have been under the care of an allergist, usually return to normal when their carbohydrate intakes are controlled. Stuffy noses clear up and, in the baby, diaper rashes vanish. One baby made a dramatic response when he was taken off fruits and tapioca pudding—high sources of carbohydrates. His diaper rash began to disappear as if by magic.

My experience has shown that a program of carbohydrate control takes care of from 50 to 60 percent of these suspected allergy cases. A number of children felt better and seemed less nervous when they were taken off milk. If a child does not improve, he should then go to an allergist.

It is especially important to emphasize, in preventing allergy, that a *variety* of good foods should be eaten. Very often, when a reaction to food occurs, it is to a food which is predominantly consumed, often to the exclusion of others. For instance, it is important to get a variety of

103

protein foods and the diet should include beef, fowl, fish, cheeses and legumes—not merely beef all the time. Eating a mixture of the basic foods together, rather than one continually by itself, is also a more logical way to do it.

The sooner these nonspecific "allergies" are tackled, of course, the better it is for the child. Lawrence's case reflects how one case of masquerading "allergies" responded to orthomolecular pediatrics.

At eighteen months of age, Lawrence suffered from recurring diarrhea, diaper rashes, face rashes, a perpetually runny nose, itchy eyes, and overactivity. Was Lawrence allergic? Certainly, except for one thing: food and milk elimination procedures helped not a bit. Indeed, at one leading Eastern medical center an intestinal tube had been passed down and a piece of Lawrence's intestinal lining was snipped out and studied for a deficiency of the enzyme lactase, which digests the milk sugar lactose. Tests showed Lawrence had a lactase deficiency, all right, but treatment for it didn't end his diarrhea.

Because careful workups had already been done, ruling out specific organic causes, when Lawrence was brought to me I ordered a five-hour glucose tolerance test. The results were revealing. Lawrence's highs and lows on the five-hour curve were quite erratic and offered an insight into how Lawrence was reacting to an overload of carbohydrates.

Lawrence's mother was advised to keep a diet diary for a week on her son and then, becoming acquainted with every element involved, to start cutting down his overall carbohydrate intake. She was taught how to get rid of all sucrose. Processed baby foods—for even the meats may have sugar added—were to be replaced by baby food made from home-grinding of meats and raw vegetables. Then Lawrence was limited to 60 grams of complex carbohydrates per day, which should have been about perfect for his age and growth needs.

Milk was eliminated and Lawrence was given a digestive enzyme of pancreatic extract, which would improve further digestion of protein and contribute to a more stable blood sugar. He was too young to swallow tablets, so he was put on a sugarless liquid vitamin complex twice a day; large amounts of vitamin C (two teaspoons twice a day of a liquid containing 300 milligrams to the teaspoon) and a complete vitamin formula that also contained members of the B-complex family not usually found in commercial products, including PABA, choline, inositol, and biotin. Calcium and phosphorus supplements were added to compensate for his having no milk.

The colds continued intermittently for six weeks, but after two months Lawrence was having normally-formed stools for the first time in his life. He went from having four or five bowel movements a day to only one. His "allergies" had cleared up, and he was less agitated.

Eight months later, Lawrence reappeared in the office with colds, diarrhea, and excitability. Questioning revealed Lawrence's carbohydrate overload had returned, in the form of fruits and ice cream. When the consequences of this deviation from the program were linked to Lawrence's revived symptoms, his father vowed to keep this in mind thereafter.

Psychosomatic Complaints

A "psychosomatic illness" is a label in search of a disease. In practice, "psychosomatic" tends to mean that the trouble can't be diagnosed as a specific organic disorder. It is as if a catch-all bag were supplied to hold all the symptoms that won't fit neatly somewhere else.

Psychosomatic complaints are often expressed as aches and pains in various parts of the body, headaches, nausea, or car sickness. When a thorough physical examination reveals no organic cause for the complaints, they are frequently termed psychosomatic. The diagnosis is saying, in effect, to the patient, "It's all in your mind." The psychological effect on the patient, upon learning "there's nothing wrong with you," is certain to be disturbing. Some may feel guilty to have bothered the doctor with "nothing." Others are left with self-doubts, wondering about the accuracy of their own feelings, perhaps even suspecting something is wrong mentally. This may be especially difficult for children when an authority figure like a doctor announces, "I can't cure you—it's all in your head."

Such an approach doesn't have to be used, though. Obviously, there is *something* wrong, whether the examination reveals it or not. To the patient the symptoms are real and affect his sense of well-being. A better way is to recognize the problems as existing, by explaining that the symptoms—once organic causes have been ruled out by a thorough examination and tests—are psychochemical. "It's in the chemistry in your head, not in your thinking." The child then better understands his problem, may even be relieved, and is in a position to cooperate actively in his treatment.

Psychosomatic symptoms are forms of an irritable nervous system and can be seen on five-hour glucose tolerance tests. When erratic up-and-down curves occur in the test, it is very common for the child to have had psychosomatic complaints of pain in various parts of the body. This becomes more understandable when we realize that these up-and-down blood sugar curves are laboratory indications of what the child is experiencing in his nervous system: a jangling disruption of smooth neural transmissions that could have an impact almost anywhere in the body.

The first step, nutritionally, is the same as in most

instances of dietary imbalance: eliminate caffein, sugar and other refined carbohydrates, and limit even complex carbohydrates.

Drugs and Alcohol

"Street" drugs—marijuana, cocaine, heroin, amphetamines or "speed", and others—are a serious problem with teen agers today, and many addicts are introduced to drugs even in elementary school. In addition, the National Institute on Alcohol Abuse and Alcoholism has estimated that there are *1.3 million* preteens and teen agers in this country with serious drinking problems. Some of these problem drinkers started as young as eight and nine years of age.

There are two ways in which eating habits may be relevant to these problems.

1. Malnutrition can make children more susceptible to street drugs because they don't feel well.

2. Proper nutrition can aid recovery during treatment for drug abuse.

Stress has an impact upon the endocrine system, especially upon the adrenals, and may lead to desire for artificial stimulation. Low blood sugar is a consistent laboratory finding in drug addicts and alcoholics. On glucose tolerance tests their blood sugars frequently dip into the 40s after three hours. In a search to feel better—physiologically, to raise the blood sugar—most children turn to caffein and sugar. Others, however, depending on their social environment and the influence or example of others, may choose street drugs or alcohol for the same purpose. By building up the child's body so that he can better withstand stress, you may be able to help head off these crises in many instances.

Once drug addiction or alcohol abuse has afflicted the

child, psychological counseling will be needed, but the patient will have to be motivated to want to stop using drugs or alcohol. Nutrition is a recovery tool; without motivation it is useless. But in the properly motivated patient, nutrition can start helping the body rebuild itself and can help improve the child's sense of well-being so that a relapse into addiction is less likely.

The Hospitalized Child

Some children will require more than "better nutrition" to get well. A doctor's care will be essential. In other cases, the child may have to be hospitalized. In either instance, nutrition is of the utmost importance as a means of supportive therapy. As Hans Selye states, "the least physicians and dieticians can do is to see to it that the person they are treating is not burdened with the additional stress of food nutritionally deficient or tasteless. Good food may not hasten a patient's recovery, but poor food certainly induces stress that can delay it."

Unfortunately, resistance foods are not always emphasized in hospital kitchens. Usually, a tactful conference with the physician will enable the parent to have an influence over the type of foods that will appear on her child's tray. If the physician is nutrition-oriented, there should be little problem. The parent, though, is in a position to see whether the meals contain sugars and refined starches, and can bring any accidental deviation in diet to the attention of the proper person. Certainly the parent can guard against sweets or "treats" being brought into the hospital room by well-meaning friends or relatives.

The Parents' Role: A Case History

The cases of DiAnna and her brother Paulie are good

examples of what can be done by parents to improve their children's health. Although both cases were under medical supervision, they indicate the highly significant part parents can play by "merely" seeing that their children are on a proper dietary program, primarily one of carbohydrate control and promotion of recovery foods such as protein and vitamins. It will be seen that drugs, though sometimes necessary in pediatric medicine, played a minimal role in returning the children to health.

The cases of DiAnna and Paulie, both chronically sick children, also illustrate how similar health problems tend to occur within a single family, and they point to a pattern: the degree of success depends largely upon the parents' belief in the program and their cooperation.

DiAnna was nearly three when her mother first brought her in. She cried constantly—"around the clock," her mother testified—and from birth had suffered colic, an acute abdominal pain which afflicts many babies. She had had the works: loose stools, diaper burn, bronchitis. Another pediatrician had put DiAnna on soy milk for her "milk allergy" and had assured the parents that she would outgrow the colic.

Yet DiAnna seemed to have a stomach ache all of the time and was fretful and restless. Periodically she would alternate between diarrhea and constipation, which in an older individual would have been a possible sign of colon cancer. She also experienced frequent urination which is a possible sign of diabetes.

Diabetes was ruled out by a glucose tolerance test. Indirect physiologic evidence indicates her frequent urination may have been related to a high carbohydrate diet which causes fluid retention in the body; this could contribute to the urinary problem. Excitement of the central nervous system also can be a factor in a "nervous bladder."

Among the suspect items of DiAnna's diet were apple

109

juice, orange juice, cereals, canned peaches and mixed fruit (all contained added sugar), lollipops, soda pop, colas, marshmallow whip, natural honey, and occasional coffee and tea, which she definitely liked, according to her mother. In addition, DiAnna disliked vegetables and meats.

It seemed clear that DiAnna was suffering from an overload of refined carbohydrates, with a further complication of caffein intake. Because of her age and weight, her carbohydrate limit was set at 60 grams per day. In addition to cutting her sugar and caffein consumption to as close to zero as possible, protein meals and snacks were ordered, along with vitamins—liquid C, B-complex, and a complete formula. The purpose of these supplements to her diet was to stabilize her blood sugar, by making up for any deficiencies she may have developed.

It was also necessary to describe carefully the complex carbohydrate foods that DiAnna could eat, for her mother had by now explained, "we don't eat sweets." She did not realize how widespread refined carbohydrate foodstuffs are; that the soda pop, cereals, canned fruit, and honey were loaded with sugar.

When she first returned two an a half months later, DiAnna's mother reported, "She's a different child." DiAnna had more energy and a healthy glow to her face. She still had mild stomach disorders, but 95 percent of her bowel movements were normal, a marked improvement.

Her mother also had discovered another intricate relationship between diet and her daughter's health: DiAnna no longer had any urinary urgency unless she exceeded her daily carbohydrate limit of 60 grams. The physiological explanation of this pleasant side effect is involved; the important thing to the patient and the parent is that help was offered and not withheld, as is so often the case with nutritional problems.

Several months later, DiAnna suffered what seemed to be a relapse. One night she had a nightmare and during the day she had erupted into a temper tantrum that was almost a seizure. She repeatedly disobeyed her parents and, again, she was having to urinate frequently.

The program at this point had to be reexamined. Dolomite, a good source of magnesium, was added to the regimen (78 milligrams of magnesium per tablet, one taken twice a day). She was to take 600 milligrams of vitamin C twice a day. A sugarless source of liquid B vitamins was prescribed, just in case she was getting enough from her vitamin tablets to cause the trouble. (Chewable vitamins for children are usually sweetened for taste.) For the time being, dilantin (*Infa-Tab*, 50 milligrams twice a day), a drug that often quiets children who have seizure-like outbursts of temper, was added. A major effect of dilantin is to raise the blood sugar. (The doses used for behavior disorders in children would be small enough to preclude the many side effects of the massive dosages used in epileptics. Dilantin does deplete the body of folic acid and vitamin B_6, and probably of certain minerals like zinc, but this would be compensated for by the vitamin therapy used in any good nutritional program.)

Vitamin C doses as high as those given DiAnna should be supervised by a doctor, even though no known harmful effects of large doses of vitamin C have been reported in children anywhere. Dr. Fred Klenner, a physician-researcher in Reidsville, North Carolina, has never reported any harmful effects after using large doses in all age groups over the past twenty-five years. There is, however, a harmless acid irritation effect on the urethra in some susceptible people, just as if they were exposed to the acids of soap, bubble bath agents, coffee, tea, colas, or martinis. In some children, doses over 500 milligrams per day—because it may make them feel like urinating—can aggravate enuresis (bedwetting) or simulate it, and needlessly alarm the unsuspecting parent.

A month later DiAnna seemed happier, and her mother felt that the dolomite definitely helped. But DiAnna was having trouble keeping her carbohydrate limit at 60 grams, and she still tried to drink tea.

DiAnna showed slow steady progress; by the end of a year's treatment her mother reported she was "doing very well," free of urinary frequency and less nervous. Most important of all, now—at age four—she had become free of colds and bronchitis. This meant the family budget was spared the usual high American bills for antibiotics.

At this point DiAnna—who had gained two pounds and grown two inches during the previous four months, a good record—was allowed 85 grams of high-quality carbohydrates daily, more in line with her increased growth and increased energy needs. At her next checkup she was taken off dilantin, which she no longer needed. She was doing fine.

It was now fifteen months after her initial visit and she had reached a point where she could definitely be pronounced "in good health." The same phrase could have been used many months before, but now there would be no doubt of the program's success. Nothing had happened quickly, but there it was in the words of DiAnna's mother:

"Basically, she's very, very normal, and happy all day. She leaves me alone, unless she gets the wrong kind of carbohydrates, such as a lollipop, or perhaps too high in total carbohydrates.

"She has a great deal of patience. Before, she shrieked daily. I didn't think anything would be left of her mentally because she was so nervous."

Her brother Paulie, who was seven when his mother

first brought him in, suffered from frequent episodes of cramps, vomiting, sore throat, and loose bowel movements. He would turn white periodically and become weak and exhausted. Weight losses sometimes followed. He also had suffered chronically from stomach aches and had violent headaches.

Paulie's glucose tolerance test provided a dramatic insight into the struggle going on inside him. Instead of peaking at 160 milligrams percent after one hour, Paulie's zoomed to *258* within *30 minutes*. Then it plummeted nearly as sharply as it had risen, after which it zigzagged erratically until starting downhill in the later hours. (See Paulie's curve in Figure 4–1.)

To regulate his erratic blood sugar, which may have indicated a prediabetic tendency, Paulie followed a more–or–less routine carbohydrate control program, with protein six times a day—at each meal and a small snack between meals and before going to bed.

Six weeks later, when Paulie returned for a checkup, the results made both his mother and me beam.

"He has so much more stamina!" his mother said. "He plays and walks vigorously, and his teacher and coach said he's a whole new person."

In some cases, the approach used with Paulie may work well for a while, then prove less effective. In such instances, a special low fat and low cholesterol diet that is also relatively low in protein and high in complex carbohydrates often will prove helpful. Recent evidence indicates that a high protein diet from animal sources also is high in fat and contains too much fat for many children.

Although, as I have noted, a drug may have to be prescribed for short term use to help the patient get well faster, nutritional innovations are the long range factors that have the more lasting effects. At the heart of the success of these cases was coöperation at home. The

Figure 4-2. Paulie's Glucose Tolerance Test

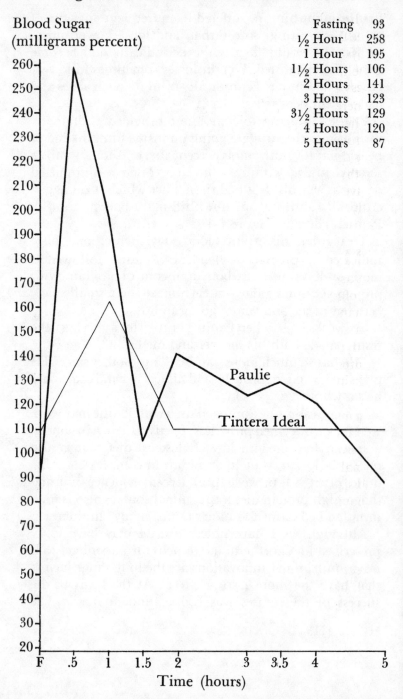

Blood Sugar
(milligrams percent)

Fasting	93
½ Hour	258
1 Hour	195
1½ Hours	106
2 Hours	141
3 Hours	123
3½ Hours	129
4 Hours	120
5 Hours	87

Paulie

Tintera Ideal

Time (hours)

implications are clear. If a child is sick, he should be taken to see the doctor. But the parents can insure that the child enjoys sound nutrition, whether he is sick or healthy. If he is well, it can help him remain that way. Prevention of illness begins at home—in the kitchen.

There is also another implication. If you can improve the health of a child with nutrition, you will usually improve his behavior and scholastic performance at the same time. It happens over and over again. If the child is healthy and enjoys a stable supply of blood sugar, he will behave normally; when this occurs he can learn more easily.

Does a Sick Child "Catch Up"?

Let's assume that a child responds to nutrition and "snaps out of it." He regains his color, energy, vigor, and resistance. But what of the "lost" months and years? Will he or she ever be able to make up for that?

On the basis of work with malnourished Peruvian children, there are indications that a dramatic improvement in the child's nutrition may enable him to "catch up." The children studied were those who had suffered from malnutrition in the slums of Lima, Peru. Taken to a superior home environment, with regular meals and improved hygiene, the children seemed to not only resume normal growth but to make up by gaining in height and head size. Although this study related to the malnutrition of poverty, a victim of the malnutrition of affluence should be able to recover similarly.

However, even when a child perks up almost immediately on an improved diet, it does not follow that he is in perfect health. In the child's cells, down at the molecular level, all of the damage is not so swiftly repaired. Dr. Roger J. Williams has stated that it takes from three to five

115

years to rebuild the body to a state of homeostasis (biochemical balance) under stress. However, acceptable improvement in treated cases of behavior disorders and learning problems will occur within four to six weeks, sometimes as soon as ten days. Recovery from low resistance to infections is slower; it may take two to three months or longer. This means recovery of health through nutrition may be slower than a parent wishes. In cases of slow improvement, it is often encouraging to periodically compare the child's condition *now* with what it was *then*, before his diet was altered.

In sum, nutrition is a vital factor in illness and health. Proper fueling of the human machine helps prevent illness by maintaining health. When illness has occurred, nutrition should become a tool aiding in recovery. Just as importantly, a long-term nutritional program is a necessity following an illness. The fact that the child seems well and has recovered from the obvious clinical manifestations of a disorder does not mean that all of the body's chemistry is automatically back in order—that takes time. This is perhaps the strongest argument there is for the use of a nutritional program that will help build resistance and thereby prevent sickness.

Psychological Tips

In changing the dietary routine, the child should be granted the privilege of making some of his own decisions about food and eating—within careful limits. *He should not be forced to eat.* If he is not interested in food at one meal, he should be allowed to leave the table. But once having decided to pass up the opportunity to eat, he must also learn that his decision is final—another opportunity to eat will not arrive until the next meal. In time, the youngster learns that eating is a privilege and not a duty.

The child also learns that it is fun to be hungry enough to want to eat, a delight that becomes more apparent to him when he does not eat, drink, or chew anything between meals or designated snacktimes.

The establishment of regular meal times can be very helpful. This regularity aids in calming the excitable child and allows sufficient time between meals for an appetite to develop. Limiting all sources of excitement for fifteen or twenty minutes before meals is also helpful, since it causes loss of interest in food. Finally, a pleasant atmosphere at the table is always conducive to good digestion. Unpleasant arguments and harsh remarks, of any kind, frighten little children into losing interest in food. Children of all ages thrive on laughter and this is the best table atmosphere for them.

Good eating habits don't come from tonics in bottles. They have to be taught. Without them, no amount of vitamin B_{12}, iron, thiamine, or anything else will make a child eat.

Most of all, *both* parents must be united on the carbohydrate control program if it is to work for the child. If one parent insists on a sugarless diet and on limiting total carbohydrates, while the other allows or "rewards" the child with an ice cream cone, soda pop, or a candy bar, the child can't be expected to get well. One parent is sabotaging the good work the other is doing. Coöperation is essential in all phases of the child's nutritional program.

What You Can Do to Improve Your Child's Health

1. If your child has severe tonsillitis or any other chronic or infectious disorder, take him to a doctor. *Do not attempt to treat serious disorders without medical attention.*

2. Attempt to find a doctor who is interested in the nutritional approach. If unable to find one already so oriented, then try to get your physician interested.

3. While following the doctor's prescription on emergency medication aimed at eradicating symptoms, start the child on the carbohydrate control program by eliminating dietary sugar and all *refined* carbohydrates *completely*. But you should include nutritious carbohydrates such as whole grains (bread, rice, and cereal), fruits (moderately), vegetables, and legumes such as peas and beans.

4. For the small child, in addition to the other parts of the program, follow this schedule:

UNDER ONE YEAR:

Restrict fruits and juices to no more than 2 oz. once a day—always with food.

"Practice" foods started at two to three months must all be pureed. All solid foods should remain pureed until the child is eighteen months old. (A child under eighteen months old may choke on coarse food; his chewing motions are also imperfect for properly grinding food until the age of two-and-one-half years.)

At three to six months start whole grain cereals, bread or crackers and vegetables. Start pureed meat, fish, or chicken three times a day in *small* anounts, to avoid overloading the kidneys.

No processed baby foods with sugar, additives, coloring, or flavoring.

No desserts or cold drinks.

ONE TO SIX YEARS:

In addition to the above, limit milk to 16 to 24 ounces a day.

118

5. If the child has no health problems requiring medical attention, then start him on the carbohydrate control program anyway. Cut out all sugar, whether from soda pop, candy, ice cream, or desserts, and all refined starches found in white flour products and cereals. (However, in order to insure the cooperation of some children it may be necessary to substitute carob syrup, tupelo low-sugar honey, or artificial sweeteners in recipes. The quantity should be carefully regulated.)

6. Remove *all* forms of caffein from the diet, whether it's from colas (including *Dr. Pepper*), root beer, chocolate, tea, or coffee.

7. Make certain the child is getting a sufficient daily supply of protein, such as an egg or a serving of meat, chicken, or fish at each meal. If he seems to show fatigue, *small* protein snacks of cheese, nuts, or meats should be given between meals. Protein servings need not be large; quality is more important than quantity.

8. Insure that he is receiving his daily quota of foods from the Four Basic Groups—meats (and vegetable protein), dairy products, vegetables and fruit, and breads and cereals. Use whole grain bread and cereals instead of the "enriched," refined ones, and buy unsweetened, unhydrogenated peanut butter, the natural kind.

9. Use these limits as a guide to carbohydrate control in children and make certain that all the carbohydrates are starches:

Small children to the age of two, 50-60 grams
Three to six, 75-100 grams; milk to 16-24 ounces daily
Six to eight, 100-115 grams
Eight to ten, 120-135 grams
Ten to thirteen, 135-150 grams

Teen agers may require more than 150 grams, depending on their size and energy needs and how fast they are growing, but a need for more than 250 grams of carbohydrates per day is unusual—such a large amount might be needed by an older teen-aged, massive athlete.

10. If your child should be hospitalized for any reason, do everything you can, *tactfully*, to see that his diet there is high in resistance foods and contains no harmful foods or drinks.

11. Most of all, remember that healthful nutrition is a daily habit that must be acquired. This means you will have to become conscious *every day* of what you and your child are eating. To maintain health, you will have to maintain a high level of nutrition. Eternal vigilance is the price of health!

12. Finally, parents should change their own diets. The best way to encourage proper eating habits in your child is to set a good example.

5

"Why Doesn't He Behave?"

At thirteen, Arthur seemed to be "worrying himself sick" over the most ordinary events, when he should have been out playing with other children. Often his temper would build up and erupt. "Things just get on my nerves," he explained. His unpredictable emotional outbursts shocked those around him.

Unusual behavior stood out in Arthur's case, though there were other factors in his overall health picture that were just as important. Invariably there is more than one symptom when a child has problems. Arthur was also noticeably obese—178 pounds on a five-foot-nine-inch frame. The massive, stocky youngster also suffered severe headaches every three or four weeks and when he flexed his knee sharply, severe cramps seized his hamstring muscles.

However, his behavior—seeming to be a psychochemical aberration—was the element that nudged his parents

121

into taking Arthur to the doctor. As I examined him, I noted his rigid movements. His truculent facial expression pulled his mouth leftward. He endured the examination with sweating, jerking, and apprehension, all physical signs of psychological stress.

As I studied his medical history I learned that as a small child he had suffered bloating from drinking too much milk and had had bronchitis from time to time. He had also experienced some allergies. More recently, he had been concerned about his tendency to gain weight.

Next I looked into his nutritional background.

BREAKFAST—Egg and bacon, orange juice and toast.

MORNING SNACK—*Cola* and *candy*.

LUNCH—Ham-and-cheese sandwich, fruit, and *cake, cookies*, and milk.

AFTERNOON SNACK—*Cola*, milk.

DINNER—Seconds on *sweets*, with hefty servings of milk and *sugared tea*.

First impressions pointed toward imbalances in both carbohydrate intake and vitamins. A five-hour glucose tolerance test was ordered. Arthur's blood sugar curve, shown in Figure 5-1, did not at any time approach the ideal standard. It remained below ideal levels throughout the test. This told us why he ate so much—trying futilely to boost his blood sugar, so he'd feel better. His fondness for between-meal snacks of cola drinks and candy was also explained.

Arthur's therapy began with the usual carbohydrate control program, tailored to his age and special needs:

Sugar: none.

Complex carbohydrate limit: 115 grams per day. (This was lower than usual for a boy his age, in order to achieve weight reduction.)

Protein: Six times a day (at meals and snacks).

Figure 5-1. Arthur's Glucose Tolerance Test

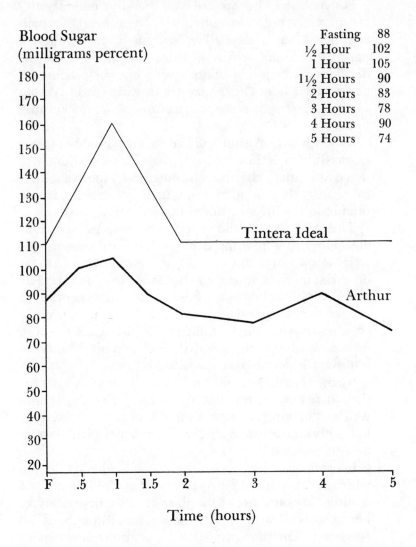

Blood Sugar
(milligrams percent)

Fasting	88
½ Hour	102
1 Hour	105
1½ Hours	90
2 Hours	83
3 Hours	78
4 Hours	90
5 Hours	74

Tintera Ideal

Arthur

Time (hours)

For Arthur I also prescribed a digestive enzyme, a B-complex vitamin formula, and a general vitamin capsule: twice a day. (The enzyme is an extract of pancreatic tissue which elevates the blood sugar by digesting protein. There are several enzyme products of pancreatic origin. Other enzymes are different and do not work as effectively as the pancreatic enzymes in handling protein.)

A month later, Arthur had had only one mild headache, no ear fluid, was thinner (having lost 13 pounds), and was much more alert, cheerful, and outgoing. His psychological rigidity, brooding, and outbursts had receded in one brief month with nutritional therapy alone.

Thereafter, Arthur did experience "relapses" occasionally. Once, five months later, after he had brought his weight down 26 pounds, to 152, he grew too nervous to eat breakfast in the morning and his hands would shake. His carbohydrate ceiling was raised to 150 grams per day, to take care of greater energy needs. From time to time he checked in with other problems—a bad headache once, nausea another time, a football injury to his shoulder—but overall his progress was evident.

By the time he was fifteen, close to two years after his first office visit, Arthur was "doing fine." He was sleeping well and making A's and B's in school. He seemed to be just a normal teenaged boy, probably better than normal, because of his diet.

Behavior problems vary with the individual child and with age. Perhaps a little kindergarten child, instead of cutting out dolls, throws the gluepot on the floor, tears up her neighbor's work, and wreaks havoc throughout the classroom. One day, the school's administrator gets in touch with the mother: "You must come and get her. You'll just have to keep her at home!" Or let's say the child is a twelve-year-old. His behavior was pleasant enough two years ago, but now he is brutally rude, irritable and he stays up half the night and sleeps all day. Or maybe the mother enters her early teenager's bedroom to find him on the floor with an empty bottle of pills beside him.

In any case, the psychological factors must always be considered—especially the possibility of a breakdown in family relations. But in behavior cases I have handled, there is more involved. In most instances, the problems seemed to be more physiological than psychological, or a mixture of the two.

Blood Sugar and Behavior

What these problem children may have in common, from the pre-schooler to the distraught, despair-filled teen ager, is the failure of a malnourished brain to right itself under stress. Despite whatever else is involved, the malnutrition of affluence seems to have inflicted behavior difficulties upon a large portion of our children. Unstable blood sugar is usually a crucial key to these problems.

As one authority on diabetes, Dr. Guy Lacy Schless, has pointed out, a rapid blood sugar drop can bring on classic hypoglycemic (low blood sugar) symptoms: sweating, pallor, confusion, difficulty focusing the eyes, headaches. In some people these symptoms can appear with relatively minor blood sugar changes, as when the blood sugar drops from, say, 140 to 70 milligrams percent, traditionally considered "within normal ranges."

When the child's blood sugar is unstable or remains too low, some of the same symptoms of hypoglycemia may be felt, even though he would not be classified as hypoglycemic by the usual criteria. In some persons, such symptoms may mimic psychoses. Drs. Gilles Lortie and Dean M. Laird, psychiatrists at the Worcester State Hospital in Massachusetts, have noted such disorders of the central nervous system to include the "inability to speak properly, purposeless movements, incoördination, silliness, negativism, twitching, incoherence, and mental dullness." They went on to say that these symptoms have at times been improperly diagnosed as epilepsy, alcoholism, brain tumor, anxiety neurosis, hysteria, and psychosis.

Investigators have noted over the decades that psychological disturbance is one of the characteristic signs of nutritional deficiencies resulting from stress. In studies of severely malnourished children, apathy and irritability were evident; as pointed out by Dr. Herbert G. Birch and Joan Dye Gussow in their careful study, *Disadvantaged Children*, severely ill children seemed to lose their natural curiosity. These cases, invariably, were those of severe protein-calorie malnutrition. The malnutrition of affluence does not necessarily cause protein-calorie deficiency, but it does bring on other problems that have just as striking effects on behavior. Research has linked psychological disorders with nutritional deficiencies. These behavioral studies, related to diet, have ranged from observations on schizophrenia to alcoholism. One of medicine's classic examples is that of the often severe mental disorders related to pellagra which is caused by a nutritional deficiency in niacin, or vitamin B_3. Just as much as adults, children need niacin, a stable blood sugar, and the other nutrients necessary for both healthy minds and bodies. The malnutrition of affluence might be called a *quality* deficiency disease.

A prominent psychologist, Dr. Josef Brožek, once commented, "Deficiency of all of the major nutrients, including water, eventually affects behavior even though the mechanisms involved will vary."

The body's chemical stabilizing mechanism is of greatest significance. The closer the child's blood sugar curve on the GTT comes to 100–110 milligrams percent, which is within the "ideal" range, the more improvement can be expected in his behavior. (With the homeostasis blood sugar test, however, during which the patient eats as usual during the testing, the blood sugar never goes above 85 or below 75 in persons with normal physiology who are eating and drinking properly. These different figures on the two tests may be considered comparable, for the measurements are reached by different techniques with which to measure the different components.) In the same way that infections are fought or prevented by increasing resistance foods while deleting susceptibility foods, improper behavior can often be corrected or at least helped. Nutritional imbalance in a child is likely to result in nervous irritability. The same solid nutrition that wards off the stress of disease will also help prevent environmental stress by improving the brain's ability to withstand irritation. It is often necessary for me to explain to the child, "Your problems with Mother and Dad won't go away, but you'll be able to deal with them better when your nutrition improves."

Bedwetting is one of the biggest unsolved neurological problems in pediatrics. There is no satisfactory treatment. I have never seen bedwetting cured with nutrition, but I have seen some patients improve over a period of time when their nutrition was optimal, after other efforts had failed. Bedwetting is one case, however, in which added vitamin C supplements can make the problem worse; the excess of the vitamin goes through the kidney and collects in the bladder, where it is enough of an irritant to cause the child to want to urinate.

On the other hand, another so-called problem—thumb sucking—is not really a behavioral problem. The baby is born with the ability, instinct, and desire to suck. Any dental harm usually disappears before any permanent damage can be done. Many parents have been driven into a frenzy of corrective actions: adhesive tape, bandages, quinine, turpentine. If your young child sucks his thumb, leave him alone.

In fact, the late Dr. Leo Kanner, one of the world's foremost child psychiatrists, saw more patients in his practice who had been made nervous wrecks by parental efforts to stop thumbsucking than he did cases caused by dental malocclusion. However, in the school-age child some dental harm could occur. As the dental authorities Drs. Maury Massler and Arthur W.S. Wood have noted "thumbsucking above the age of six is not to be viewed as casually as in younger children."

Now let us look at more serious behavior disorders and what may be early clues to their development, especially as they relate to hyperactivity. The range of behavior problems is quite wide. Some of them begin in the earliest years. Most children with improper behavior are hyperactive to varying extents. To give an overall idea of how undesirable behavior may develop in children, let's examine the subject by several stages of growth.

Prebirth

Many mothers of hyperactive children state that the baby kicked more in the uterus than normal children.

Infancy (Birth to Two Years)

1. Colic (frantic crying for no known reason) is the number–one symptom of hyperactivity in later life.
2. Overeating starts. The comfortable baby won't eat much.
3. Colicky babies are constantly fed to quiet them. Habits of obesity may begin here.

4. Unusual sleepiness in the newborn may be the first sign of hypoglycemia.

5. Very early motor developments such as rolling over, sitting, walking, and frantic running are early signs of hyperactivity.

Preschool (Two-Five Years)

1. Hyperactivity, whether caused by genetic, congenital, or psychochemical factors, may begin at this age.

2. The "spastic butterfly"—the child who revs up at 90 miles-per-hour as if connected to 220 volts—makes his appearance at this age.

3. Destructiveness develops; the child's interest in books is likely to consist of throwing them or tearing pages.

4. Rages and temper tantrums begin.

5. Sleep resistance disrupts his schedule.

6. Withdrawal from, or abusiveness toward, peers characterizes his relationships.

7. If control of eating habits is not accomplished by this point, the malnutrition of affluence and further hyperactivity can be expected.

Early School Years (Six to Fourteen Years)

1. Hyperactivity of a nonorganic cause may begin here as a reaction to the first grade, especially if the child has any learning disabilities or visual and coördination problems.

2. School problems may make some children moody.

3. Boisterousness, to an excess, may occur.

4. Overtalkativeness.

5. Disruptive, inappropriate fears appear in reaction to

129

school problems. Often the child may be branded as lazy, a day-dreamer, stupid, rebellious, as a result.

Later School Years, Puberty

1. In extreme cases, running away from home sometimes occurs.
2. In the older child, physical hyperactivity may be replaced by a disruptive argumentative personality.

Although this developmental scheme gives us some clues to watch out for, it may not necessarily fit every child who presents behavior difficulties. Most of all, it provides a *general* guide so that the parent can see a pattern and then intervene before the problem worsens. It can also be a stimulus to place the child on a nutritional program to help prevent any possibility of such problems appearing later.

Based upon my own experience, I am inclined to classify hyperactivity into three types:

1. That which has its onset at birth, with overreactive shaking and crying in the newborn infant. This seems to be genetic in origin (congenital) or associated with birth trauma.
2. That which starts at around two to four years of age. It is probably caused by nutritional imbalance of some kind (high carbohydrates, nutrient deficiency) or allergy. Although some suspicions have been aroused as to the relationship between bottle feeding, with its high sugar content, and hyperactivity, this has not yet been studied in depth.
3. That hyperactivity which starts at school age and is the child's response to learning problems, related to visual and hearing difficulties.

Whatever the cause or the type, improvement is practically always possible. The case of Mitch, who was almost five, illustrates how early intervention can avoid a lot of problems later on. Mitch frequently had erections and masturbated in public. As if this weren't embarrassment enough to his parents, he also was rebellious, struck his playmates and screamed belligerently. Around adults, he was a nuisance. Everyone asked: "Why doesn't he behave?"

Mitch had no apparent deficiencies. He was getting more than enough protein. But he was consuming too much sugar—26 teaspoons of *actual* sugar daily, contained in food and drink, plus the equivalent of 55 teaspoonsful of sugar from refined carbohydrates—and even more importantly, his total carbohydrate intake amounted to a staggering overload. Instead of the 80 grams of complex carbohydrates he should have been taking, he was swallowing 320 grams a day, four times too much.

Mitch's five-hour glucose tolerance test (Figure 5-2) exhibited an up-and-down pattern, with a 69–milligram drop in the third hour. With his blood sugar behaving like that, how could Mitch's actions ever be socially appealing?

Placed on the carbohydrate control program, Mitch soon stopped masturbating. His embarrassing, disruptive behavior cleared up almost immediately. Apparently, his psychological disturbances weren't any deeper than his blood sugar.

Significantly, young children like Mitch usually respond faster to a nutritional change than do older children. This suggests that the sooner a start is made, the better the chances of success.

In instances where nutritional improvement alone does not solve the problem, the parent may be interested in trying other approaches under the direction of a physician. There are a number of other facets of

Figure 5-2. Mitch's Glucose Tolerance Test

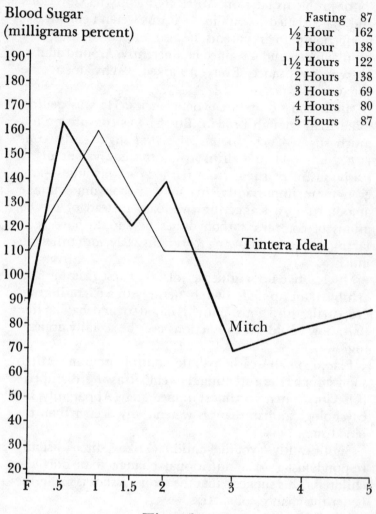

Blood Sugar
(milligrams percent)

Fasting	87
½ Hour	162
1 Hour	138
1½ Hours	122
2 Hours	138
3 Hours	69
4 Hours	80
5 Hours	87

Tintera Ideal

Mitch

Time (hours)

orthomolecular modification of behavior that may be beneficial in a particular situation. Megavitamin therapy, or high dosages, is one. Dr. Bernard Rimland of the Institute for Child Behavior Research at San Diego has reported megavitamin therapy, using vitamin C and three B vitamins (niacin, pyridoxine or B_6, and pantothenic acid), to be especially beneficial to children with severe behavior patterns, even with psychotic children. In some instances, the trouble was due to an imbalance of minerals (like potassium and calcium) and trace elements. Just as important, any buildup of toxic metals, such as lead and mercury, may lead to disturbed behavior. Dr. Allen Cott in New York has found analysis of hair samples to be an effective tool in diagnosing toxic metal levels in his work with children. Recent studies also indicate that low-level lead poisoning may be a cause of hyperactivity in children. Dr. E. K. Silbergeld of Johns Hopkins University has reported that lead-treated mice were exceedingly hyperactive—three times as much as control animals on lead-free diets.

Dr. Marshall Mandell, director of the New England Foundation for Allergic and Environmental Diseases in Norwalk, Connecticut, has demonstrated that, in certain susceptible persons, particular foods, drinks, and industrial pollutants (including fumes and automobile exhaust) may cause bizarre, otherwise inexplicable behavior patterns.

More recently, Dr. Ben F. Feingold, chief emeritus of the department of allergy at the Kaiser-Permanente Medical Center in San Francisco has reported food additives, used for artificial flavoring and coloring, are a cause of hyperactivity and learning problems in some children. There are an estimated 3,200 artificial flavors in use. More are in convenience foods than in any other form. He found that children's symptoms could be turned on and off simply by manipulating the diet in regard to additive-containing foods. His book, *Why Your Child Is Hyperactive*, is a guide to this problem. Dr. Stephen D. Lockey, Sr., an allergist in Lancaster, Pennsylvania, has prepared a list of commercial preparations that should be avoided by persons sensitive to aspirin and Dye No. 5 (tartrazine). It is a seven-page, single-spaced list of 377 commercial products by brand names and manufacturers, which gives some idea of how widely distributed the active ingredient is. For detailed information, you or your physician can write Dr. Lockey at 60 North West End Avenue, Lancaster, Pennsylvania 17603.

These additional approaches, however, do not replace the basic program of carbohydrate control. Some of these programs including those of Drs. Feingold and Lockey, do allow sugar to be used if it is not a part of one of the additive-containing foods on the avoidance list. I strongly recommend that carbohydrate control be followed in any case and that all sugar and caffein be excluded. I have found in my own practice that, no matter what other form of therapy was used, its results were closely related to the success of the carbohydrate control program, particularly the elimination of sugar and caffein.

The Hyperactive Child

Not all misbehavior is related to hyperactivity, of course, and there are even varying degrees of the problem. But there is one severe form of hyperactivity that can only be classified as extreme. The patient is one that might be called a "wild child," which may be the most difficult challenge in pediatrics today.

Life with a severely hyperkinetic (overactive) youngster is likely to be a continual nightmare. The child endlessly churns about and talks without ceasing. Eventually this unhappy child takes his toll on the entire family.

134

Unfortunately, such cases are not medical rarities. My impression is that the problem is increasing. In addition, there are many thousands of other children whose behavior doesn't quite qualify them for the "wild" category but who are edging close to the line. There is also the additional complication that, since there is no definitive medical explanation for the disorder, an improper diagnosis often results. The actual pattern of hyperactivity may vary from one child to another. Many are almost continually overactive, but some may be hyped up at school and not at home, or vice versa. Parents do not always know how to recognize the signs, and the doctor doesn't necessarily see it in the office where the child's behavior may be acceptable.

There are many puzzling aspects to hyperkinesis. Often, the overactive child stands and walks early and may learn better than the other children in the family. But he *runs*, never walks, wherever he goes. At an early age he becomes willfully antagonistic and defiant.

Hyperkinesis is usually found in children up to the age of ten. They become disruptive and can't get along with playmates. By the time such a child is five or six years old he wants to know why people don't like him. He has a very low frustration threshold. When things don't go right for him—and this is much of the time—he will throw objects in a fit of rage. By the time he reaches kindergarten he is snatching papers from other pupils, pushing and hitting them. His misplaced efforts continue into his school work. Instead of attempting to draw figures on his paper in class, he scrawls and frantically scribbles with his crayons. When you talk with his parents, you learn that their child is not getting much sleep and neither are they. Frequently the child goes on nerve-shredding behavior binges that leave the parents climbing the walls and playmates and siblings in tears.

Hyperactivity, in some cases, may persist into adult life,

but usually there is a significant change in behavior around the age of ten. The under-ten youngster is disruptive and destructive primarily through his physical actions and movements. The over-ten individual, including the teenager, is more likely to use words instead of actions, channeling his restlessness into a kind of disruptive intellectual aggression. He may hurl words instead of toys.

It was once believed that hyperkinesis was caused by brain damage, a theory that some physicians still favor. Although some cases do suggest this possibility, I feel there are other causes in the vast majority of instances. Instead of physical brain damage, which can be tested medically, in most of these patients the brain seems unable to function in an orderly manner. This is what is called a functional, rather than an organic, problem. There is no physical damage to the brain, but for some reason it is not functioning properly.

The brain has two basic functions—to activate and to inhibit or modify. As a simple example, move your hand to the window. Your hand stops at the window because your brain has performed both of its basic functions. It activated the muscles to move your hand toward the window, but the inhibitory mechanism also stopped it, or else your hand would have smashed uncontrollably through the glass. In some way the hyperactive child suffers from a breakdown of these inhibiting mechanisms. The brain doesn't balance activation and inhibition, which would allow him to operate in a smooth, normal fashion. This explains the child's ceaseless activity.

Specific problems may vary from one hyperactive child to the other. Some may have problems in speech, in balance, or perhaps in handwriting; others may perform well academically, but their behavior will be so disruptive that they can't remain in school. Their common problem

seems to be one of neural organization and function, as if
somehow the brain were being short-circuited and not
living up to its two major functions.

Based upon my own clinical experience and an
examination of the medical literature, there are a number
of potential causes of hyperactivity which should be
considered. They are as follows:

1. Intestinal parasites
2. Sugar
3. Caffein
4. Allergies
5. Salicylates (the active ingredient found in aspirin)
and food dyes that are like salicylates
6. Lead poisoning and anemia
7. Disturbed family life
8. Disturbed school environment
9. Serous otitis (an allergic or infectious middle ear
disorder) or any other cause of hearing loss
10. Visual disorders
11. Any perceptual problem, either visual or auditory,
such as a learning or reading disorder
12. Fluorescent lights or prolonged TV exposure.
Though little is known yet about either of these factors,
suspicions have been raised

Obviously, a thorough physical examination should be
conducted in such a case, in order to rule out the
possibility of overlooking some of the above problems.
Also, read labels carefully to avoid artificial coloring and
flavoring agents that may cause reactions similar to those
caused by sugar.

A medical history is also helpful in nailing down a
pattern of behavior. In my experience, the earliest clue to
the future problem usually appears shortly after birth
when the baby develops chronic colic, a nondisease, as we
said earlier, in which the baby cries frantically for no

137

apparent reason. Not all babies who have colic become hyperactive in later life, but most hyperactive children have had colic as babies.

Invariably, the parents take the colicky baby to the doctor who changes his formula, from cow's milk to a soybean derivative, based on the possibility that milk is causing the irritation. Often the baby is prescribed a calming medication, usually phenobarbital or certain stomach and intestinal relaxants. Yet because of the very immature functions of all of the homeostatic (balance) mechanisms and organs such as the liver and kidney, it is extremely dangerous to give new infants anything in excess. Even too many vitamins and minerals, which would be no problem in an older child, are risky at this age. Despite all these approaches, however, the problem baby continues to spit up food and suffer from colic during the first year of life, with nothing seeming to relieve the distress.

When the child begins walking, the signs become more noticeable. He tends to run rather than walk. At times it is difficult to tell the difference between a normally active child and a borderline hyperactive one; if you observe closely, the type of behavior will provide the key. The truly hyperactive child reacts *excessively* to his environment and, all too often, negatively. A memorable example is a five-year-old patient I saw on a weekend afternoon. He was so overactive that he had to be locked in the waiting room while I tried to talk to his mother. But he climbed through the receptionist's window twice—once when it was unobstructed and once after I set a child's rocking chair on the window sill to try to deter him. The behavior of such children is usually strikingly different from normal children. Many, for instance, will run deliberately into a wall or bang their heads on the floor repeatedly when thwarted in some desire.

A Possible Factor—Serotonin

The precise biochemical mechanism by which carbohydrate overload triggers hyperactivity is not yet spelled out. There is, however, laboratory evidence that indicates certain kinds of inappropriate behavior, including hyperactivity, are related to an imbalance in the brain of serotonin.

Serotonin (5-hydroxytryptamine) is one of several neurotransmitters in the brain. A neurotransmitter is the chemical substance in the nerve tissue responsible for communication (sending signals) from the neurons to other cells in the brain, muscle, or other parts of the body.

Serotonin is a product of the body's metabolism of the amino acid, tryptophan, but is also found in foods, especially in bananas and pineapples.

According to biochemist Dr. John J. Miller, a former editor of *Chemical Abstracts*, serotonin is essential in human metabolism, but excessive amounts in the tissues may cause toxic results. Normally, unneeded serotonin is changed into a harmless, even helpful substance. However, for this to take place the body needs adequate quantities of copper, manganese, magnesium, and vitamin B_6. Serotonin plays a vital role in the function of the central nervous system, as well as in other parts of the body. But it must be in balance with the rest of the body's chemistry. Small quantities have tranquilizing effects. A large dose excites the central nervous system and an excess in the brain may cause mental upsets. An excess, not properly handled by the body, could change into bufotenine (toad poison) or lysergic acid, which might trigger hallucinations.

The role of serotonin in children with behavior disorders has not yet been clarified. In research at St. Joseph Hospital in Lancaster, Pennsylvania, Drs. Hemmige N. Bhagavan, Mary Coleman, and David Baird

Coursin found significantly less serotonin in the blood of hyperactive children than in normal ones. In their experiment, however, no clinical study was made of its effect on the children's behavior.

Drs. John D. Fernstrom and Richard J. Wurtman, writing in *Scientific American*, have pointed out that excess carbohydrates cause a rise in serotonin in the brain, a process that begins within an hour after eating or drinking. In experiments at the Massachusetts Institute of Technology, Fernstrom and Wurtman demonstrated that insulin injections in rats increased serotonin levels in the brain. They followed this up with a carbohydrate-fat diet (without protein) which caused the body to secrete insulin naturally. Again, serotonin increased significantly in the brain in the first hour and was 20 percent above normal after two hours.

On the other hand, a high protein diet—even though it included tryptophan, the amino acid that is a precursor of serotonin—limited the uptake of tryptophan into the brain and its metabolism into serotonin. Thus, protein seems to be a stabilizing factor in the serotonin picture, and these findings with test animals seem to provide laboratory evidence of the importance of protein to the well-being of these particular children.

For very complex biochemical reasons, high carbohydrate foods caused a rise of serotonin in rats' brains. Although such precise experiments obviously can't be done with human brains, measurement of blood in human volunteers indicates the same results.

Other experiments showed that cats deprived of brain serotonin became insomniacs. Sleeplessness is often seen in hyperactive children. Other experiments indicated that rats with increased serotonin became less sensitive to pain, and there are indications in some children with special behavior problems that they are bothered much less by pain.

In other research, changes in the brain's serotonin level influenced motor activity and food consumption. "The latter finding suggests a kind of closed circle," wrote Fernstrom and Wurtman, "with food consumption affecting brain biochemistry and brain biochemistry in turn affecting food consumption ... it remains a fact that, at least in our mammalian relative the laboratory rat, diet does control the synthesis of a significant neurotransmitter. We are loath to dismiss such a finding as mere coincidence."

It is too early to say for certain what is going on in this complex relationship between serotonin levels and the rest of the body. Its role in behavior of hyperactive children has yet to be worked out in detail. Probably at some time in the near future scientists will discover that there is an ideal level of serotonin needed for the brain and nervous system. In the meantime, it is well to remember that an excess of carbohydrates in the diet may upset the balance, and this is probably why sugar upsets children so seriously. It should also be kept in mind that, specifically, copper, manganese, magnesium, and vitamin B_6 are needed in the proper amounts to metabolize any unwanted excess of serotonin. No one really knows how many other highly complex biochemical processes may be so easily disturbed in the body. The evidence we have argues very forcefully for a full, balanced diet which will supply all of the needed nutrients in the right amounts.

Treatment of Symptoms: Hyperkinesis and Drugs

At some point during treatment of severe cases the doctor, unless he is nutritionally oriented, is likely to tell the parents, "we'll have to put him on medication to calm him." Invariably, medication for the wild child means Ritalin, related to the amphetamines, which are also known as "speed".

Ritalin, paradoxically, does have a calming influence on hyperactive children—a kind of reverse effect to what might be expected in a "normal" body. The amphetamines were first used in medicine as anoretics, or appetite suppressants; they stimulated the dieting patient so that he had a sense of well-being even though he was eating much less than ordinarily. But as the amphetamine Dexedrine begin to fall into disfavor as a means of controlling obesity, it was observed that overactive children became calm with the drug, whereas the usual sedatives, such as phenobarbital, make the wild child more unruly. (Phenobarbital lowers the blood sugar; Dilantin, an antiseizure drug, raises it; the effect of Ritalin on blood sugar is not known, but it is believed to act in the body like other stimulants.) Ritalin, a derivative of Dexedrine, came to be widely prescribed for hyperkinesis.

Like most drugs, however, Ritalin has its drawbacks. While it improves the child's self-discipline to some extent, there are some patients on whom it has no effect at all, and it makes still others even worse. Large doses may cause the child to lose his appetite, become hollow-eyed, and lose weight. But once Ritalin is discontinued, the child's destructive behavior pattern reappears.

Hyperkinetic children, who live under a great deal of stress, are usually underweight to begin with. Thus it becomes distressing to use a drug that will retard growth and development, thereby aggravating an already serious situation.

Coffee has been suggested as a substitute drug in calming hyperkinetic children. The argument for this is that coffee does not produce the harmful side effects of stronger drugs. However, coffee has all of the drawbacks that Ritalin has. Any stimulant applied to the nervous system will have significant effects—the increased release of insulin, storage and release of glycogen from the liver, and stress and exhaustion upon the adrenal cortex—and all these phenomena will aggravate an unstable blood sugar condition. The caffein in coffee is a biphasic drug; that is, it has a dual nature. There may be one hour of outward benefit, but later there is a failure of auditory attention, as well as decreased efficiency in hand-eye coordination. These serious disturbances in the nervous system, to be discussed more fully in Chapter VI, are side effects that should rule out "coffee therapy" for both hyperactive and normal children.

An Alternate Approach: Nutrition

As we mentioned in the list of possible causes of hyperactivity, two suspicious factors are sugar and caffein. Any child who is hyperactive is obviously under a great deal of stress. Whatever the underlying causes of his behavior, improved nutrition can only benefit him. The elimination of sugar and caffein is of the utmost importance in managing the hyperactive child. These substances keep him hyped up and then let him down.

When following a sound nutritional program the child benefits physiologically and in most cases is likely to become self-directive and better behaved in school. The sleep pattern is usually the first sign of improvement, and the hyperkinetic will now apply himself to normal tasks. Recovery time varies from one child to the next but is usually marked by good skin color, cooperativeness, and generally quieter behavior. The child feels better.

Parents should be aware of the warning signs of extreme behavior that may indicate a hyperkinetic pattern. If they act soon enough they may be able to prevent serious problems later. Ernest's case illustrates the value of early recognition of the problem.

At age two and a half, Ernest already exhibited a severe

behavioral pattern. He was always on the go, and at night resisted going to sleep. Overly aggressive with other children, he would not respond to any kind of discipline and had to be watched constantly. His mother felt she yelled and spanked too much, but she didn't know what else to do—she was at her wit's end.

As with other children like him, Ernest had had a colicky disposition as a baby and had experienced rashes, chronic colds, tonsillitis, allergies, and diarrhea, though he was not yet three.

His overactivity could be traced from babyhood. He had been too active to diaper. As is often the case with such children, his mobility rating was high: he flipped at one month, crawled at three months, and pulled up and was creeping at six months. Ernest started walking at eight months—and he always walked *very* fast. At ten months he could climb anything in the house, and did. He spoke words at one year, sentences at fourteen months, and now could count to nine.

But along with his rapid motor and mental development there was the less pleasant side. Since eighteen months Ernest had had nightmares. He would refuse to go to sleep; his bedtime ranged from 8:30 P.M. to 12 midnight. But he always awoke at 2 A.M.—a common symptom in hypoglycemics—at which time his mother fed him. When he got up at 7 A.M. he was very irritable. Outside the house he was continually fighting with his playmates. On top of this, Ernest seemed to be totally unaware of the consequences of what he did. When scratched by a dog reacting to his behavior, Ernest continued to attack the dog. At mealtimes he would spit out his meat. He seemed driven, compelled by something over which he had no control.

Ernest's father saw his son's behavior as strictly a problem of discipline, rather than one of medicine. This is not unusual for fathers. The mother sees the child all of the time; the father usually sees him only at certain times of the day and can easily miss the seriousness of the problem. This tendency of fathers is even more pronounced in cases where the parents are separated or divorced and the father sees the child only on certain designated days and then sometimes for only a few hours.

Ernest's diet offered numerous clues to his problem.

BREAKFAST

Cereal (sugared)
Juice (all right if in controlled amounts, with food)
An egg
Toast and *jelly*
Or *cinnamon-sugar toast*

MORNING SNACK

Juice
White crackers or
Vanilla wafers

LUNCH

Vegetables
Bread and butter
Cake occasionally
Ice cream occasionally
Water or milk
(He habitually spat out his meat)

AFTERNOON SNACK

Water
Crackers (while he screamed for cookies)

DINNER

Vegetables
Oleomargarine
Water
Cake
Ice cream

The best part of it was that he sometimes ate an egg. The remainder consisted almost totally of refined carbohydrates.

Many clinicians might have thought Ernest was diabetic. (See Figure 5-3.) Blood sugar that remains above 110 milligrams percent for more than two hours is suspect as a sign of diabetes or prediabetes. Ernest's blood sugar remained above that level until the end of the fourth hour, when it dipped to 76 milligrams, then at the end of the fifth hour to 55.

Ernest was placed on a 50-gram carbohydrate limit with protein three times a day. To assist in the building-up process he would also take B-complex, C, and multiple vitamins, along with a pancreatic preparation to insure proper digestion of the protein and carbohydrates he would be getting.

One month later, Ernest's mother had good results to report.

"For the first time, he can sit down."

This was a big change in Ernest's life, wrought by manipulation of his nutrition. He still had occasional tantrums, his restless sleeping persisted, and his nose continued to be congested. An overnight cure had not been found, but a beginning had been made.

Three months later he was doing "much better." Occasional temper tantrums continued, but now he could be reasoned with. This constituted something of a major milestone. Despite an attack of tonsillitis, which was

146

Figure 5-3. Ernest's Glucose Tolerance Test

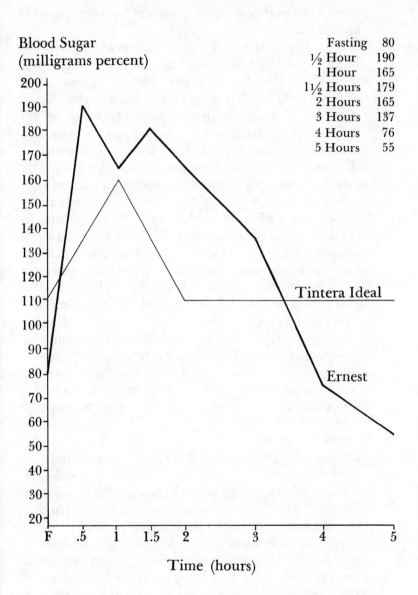

Blood Sugar
(milligrams percent)

Fasting	80
1/2 Hour	190
1 Hour	165
1 1/2 Hours	179
2 Hours	165
3 Hours	137
4 Hours	76
5 Hours	55

Tintera Ideal

Ernest

Time (hours)

treated with oral penicillin, his overall pattern reflected improvement.

Ernest, like all the other children discussed in this book, was growing. His complex carbohydrate intake was increased to 60 grams per day. He needed the added carbohydrates now that he was older, just as any normally growing child would. In hyperkinesis there is no cure *per se*. There is, at best, control. The patient is growing, becoming an adult; his case is a continuing story.

Illness is apt to bring on relapses of unwanted behavior, because of reactions to flavoring agents and sugar in the medication. This happened to Ernest, following tonsillitis. His mother phoned that he was acted wildly. In such cases it is probably best to leave the child in this agitated state until he is over the effects of his illness and the additives in his medications. Five days later she called back to report that Ernest was all right. He had settled down a good bit, but was very irritable before breakfast, a condition it took the rest of the month to reduce. (Sometimes it is possible to administer the contents of a capsule, in order to avoid the sweetener, flavoring and dye in a liquid or the coating of a tablet.)

When he was three and a half, one year after his initial visit, an examination indicated Ernest was alert, cooperative, and well-directed for his age. This was a distinct triumph for nutrition.

An overall assessment of his medical condition was: "general improvement, with periodic relapses." A persistent source of trouble to Ernest was the *concealed* sugar that entered his system. On one occasion his mother suspected a protein powder shake as the cause of her son's extreme agitation and wildness. She was right. It had been made with vanilla–flavored protein powder, egg, and milk. There probably were either sugars or additives in the protein powder to which he was sensitive. At other times

148

Ernest contributed to his own discomfort by sneaking fruits that he was not supposed to eat except with protein foods.

Despite his relapses, Ernest was a far cry from the wild child who has first visited the office a year earlier. His medical history and many others have shown us that treatment with diet and vitamins is effective in reducing hyperactivity.

As a reminder of which factors in our lives, as well as those of our children, contribute to or alleviate emotional stress, the following lists should provide some insight into what our bodies need to contend with the stresses of modern living.

NUTRITIONAL EMOTIONAL STRESS SUSCEPTIBILITY FACTORS	NUTRITIONAL EMOTIONAL STRESS RESISTANCE FACTORS
	Iron
White Flour	Iodine
Sugar and Sugar-Filled Items	Niacin
Refined Carbohydrate	Phosphorus
Substances	Animal Protein
Caffein	Vitamins B_1, B_2, B_6, B_{12}
Alcohol	Vitamins A, C, E
	Vegetable Protein
	Pantothenic Acid
	Tryptophane (Essential Amino Acid)
	Methionine (Essential Amino Acid)
	Leucine (Essential Amino Acid)
	Threonine (Essential Amino Acid)
	Phenylalanine (Essential Amino Acid)
	Potassium

Statistical Proof

A recent study of 98 of my severely hyperactive patients as a doctoral project by Ida B. Anderson in the School of Special Education and Rehabilitation at the University of Northern Colorado has confirmed that a nutritional approach is helpful in controlling hyperactivity. By feeding data from the patients' records into a computer, Anderson nailed down what had previously been observed clinically. For instance, her study demonstrated that the more hyperactive child is likely to have a gradual drop in his GTT curve, while the less hyperactive one has a sudden drop. Most important of all, this statistical analysis of the 98 patients assessed whether or not the nutritional approach influenced the children's hyperactivity. The degree of hyperactivity was rated before and after treatment by two judges, operating independently of each other. Anderson concluded in her dissertation: "The diet-vitamin treatment regimen investigated by this study was an effective treatment approach for the reduction of hyperactivity with the subject population."

Psychological Tips

Eating patterns tend to run in families, and there are indications that behavior also may run in families. Often when a hyperactive child is brought to the office, the mother will volunteer, "His daddy was like that when he was little" or "I was like that, myself." When a child craves sweets, usually there will be others in the family who tend to eat constantly. These are the "carboholics" who are hooked on refined carbohydrates just as alcoholics are on intoxicating beverages. In one family, two teenaged sisters a year apart in age displayed similar behavior problems. Both were of extremely high intelligence, one with an I.Q. of 155. When hunger struck—with blood sugar dropping—temper tantrums appeared. Both ate similar things. The family pattern extended to their mother who had hypoglycemia and suffered from fainting spells.

Likes and dislikes of foods are quite strong in some families. In pointing out the need for a resistance food like fish or eggs, I often see the mother frown and say, "His daddy doesn't like fish (or eggs), so I don't know how we're going to get him to eat it." With these children, it may be a matter of emphasizing the resistance foods that he *does* like, while later occasionally presenting the disliked foods in small quantities or as part of a dish in which it would be disguised (such as egg in a meatloaf).

Family eating patterns may extend to an entire meal. Some parents habitually skip breakfast; so do their offspring. There may be physiological reasons for this, in both instances. Many children are stimulated all day by their jitterbug diets high in caffein and sugar. At night in sleep their blood sugar may dip low. They wake up groggy in the morning, with a touch of nausea. They simply don't feel like eating, that early in the day. A child can't be expected to eat breakfast as long as his stomach is too nervous to keep the food down and digest it. He may have to continue missing breakfast until he gets better. Once his system becomes regulated, and vitamin and mineral deficiencies are made up, he will feel better in the morning. Sometimes a protein-supplement powder can be taken in lieu of breakfast by nausea-inclined children. The powder has a gelatin or bouillion-like flavor and can be mixed with liquids and drunk. It will be necessary to study the ingredients carefully, however, for some such products do have sugar in them.

Care must be taken not to antagonize the child. The parent who comes on strong with "Now, you're going to

151

do what the doctor says!'' invariably anagonizes the child. Children are led with ease but are forced with difficulty. Securing coöperation in any new regime should be approached from the viewpoint of the child himself. In what is the child interested? If the adult helps him with the problem *he's* concerned about, the way may be opened to coöperation. Often he can be shown that changing his nutritional habits will benefit him in the area of his interest. For instance, if the child likes football, a discussion of teams and of the boy's athletic achievements can lead into an explanation of how better coördination for football can result from carefully following his new diet. Properly adapted, this approach through the child's major interests could contribute to his inspired motivation.

Every age brings its own peculiar challenges. In small children, it often comes at birthday parties, with sugar and caffein galore in cake, cookies, candies, chocolate, and colas. The child shouldn't be excluded from birthday parties, for it is important he socializes with those his age. If it is his own birthday party, his mother can offer the guests wholesome snacks and drinks. There is no need to feed them sugar and caffein. If it is another child's party, it might be possible to secure the coöperation of the other mothers, so that at least your child will be offered fruit, nuts, cheese, milk or juice instead of the usual sweets. But in some cases, the mother may have to fall back on encouraging the child to eat sparingly of the risky foods and then ply him with resistance foods on arriving home. In some of these social situations, you just have to make the best of it.

The more the child understands the connection between his diet and his medical problems, the better. But since this is a complicated matter it must be made as simple as possible. I usually broach the subject something like this:

"Jacky, you know why Mom brought you here?"

"No." (guarded)

"Well, you get tired, don't you?"

"Yeah."

"And sometimes you feel funny inside?"

"Yeah." By now he usually will reflect more than a glimmer of interest.

This is a good time to show him the blood sugar curve of his five-hour glucose tolerance test, if he has taken one, comparing it with the ideal. It enables him to see the relationship between how he feels and what has happened inside him. In simple terms, he can be informed of how the blood conveys fuel to the brain in the proper amounts if he eats right and avoids the risky foods and drinks. He can be told that when he eats right, the brain receives a steady supply of fuel that will help him feel full of pep and not "funny" inside.

Delayed Treatment: A Case History

As I have said, the earlier the family recognizes behavior problems, the sooner something can be done and the better the chances of success. This does not mean nutritional changes alone, but improved nutrition should accompany whatever else is done. By the time the child becomes a teenager or young adult, all facets of treatment become increasingly difficult.

This was true in Vincent's case. At twenty-one he had been in a state hospital as well as a private psychiatric hospital. Labeled a "nervous schizophrenic," he was withdrawn and self-conscious; he felt people were watching him. He was very nervous and hyperactive.

153

At eighteen Vincent had developed suicidal tendencies and had slashed his wrists. Even as a child his hyperactivity and short attention span had necessitated supervision, for his behavior had always been erratic and undependable.

He seemed to have no self-discipline, had trouble concentrating, and wouldn't follow through with his work. Lately, he tended to sleep "all the time" and he felt he had to keep moving, a need he attributed to the sensation that people were watching him. (This may not be the reason Vincent—and other hyperactive persons like him—feel the urge to move. There is a recurring feeling of agitation that impels them to move. They have never known what it is like to feel relaxed.)

Vincent suffered from a severe anxiety neurosis; he worried incessantly about "things being wrong." He also had perceptual problems; he thought there were dust particles going into his brain and when he took a bath he felt the water in the tub was cutting him in half. These sensations may seem weird or bizarre to most people, but they are not unusual at all to schizophrenics, who through some defect fail to perceive the world as the rest of us do.

Vincent had a good intellect and usually was in good physical condition. He loved playing chess and had always like to read. But early in life he had exhibited certain symptoms that could have been clues to his future difficulties. From the time he was very small he was hyperactive. At eighteen months he was running and was always on the move. His writing had been uneven until the fifth grade; he had, in fact, printed his work until then. In examining him, I received a few more clues from his central nervous system. One of his eyelids drooped, and he seemed to be uncertain in his ideas and speech as he chatted with me.

His diet as he approached his twenty-first birthday probably offered a glimpse of what he had been consuming all his life.

BREAKFAST

Two eggs
Cereal (with sugar)
Fruit juice

MORNING SNACK

Cupcakes
Bananas
Pop tarts
Soup
Water
Milk
Cola (Through the day he drank about
3 quarts (3/4 gallon) of cola)

LUNCH

Beef or ham
Vegetable soup
Sugared tea

AFTERNOON SNACK

Cupcakes
Candy
Tea
Water
Colas

DINNER

Regular family menu, with seconds of
Pie
Cake
Tea

BEDTIME

Tea
Cupcakes

He would try to go to bed at 10 P.M. but would be up and down for an hour or so and then would sleep through until 10 o'clock the next day. He was groggy until noon. ("I hope I can stop," he said when I later pointed out the harm of caffein and sugar.)

This diet highlighted a number of serious flaws in Vincent's intake. He was getting twice the amount of protein he needed; he was eating too much of everything. But he was taking in 360 grams of carbohydrates per day, more than twice what he should have, and the wrong kind. This included 34 teaspoons of actual sugar. The additional equivalent of sugar from his refined carbohydrates amounted to another 61 teaspoons a day. A grand total of 95 teaspoons of sugar, day in, day out.

Vincent's blood sugar curve demonstrated that his fasting level was low, it then peaked too soon, and promptly plummeted to slightly below the fasting level at the 1-1/2-hour point and remained in that general range, with a somewhat jagged pattern, until the test was over. This seemed to explain why Vincent felt groggy in the mornings and why he kept snacking on sweets and consuming large quantities of sugared, caffein-laden tea and colas. The sugar and caffein represented his futile attempts to raise his blood sugar so that he could feel better. Of course, this only aggravated his situation.

Figure 5-4. Vincent's Glucose Tolerance Test

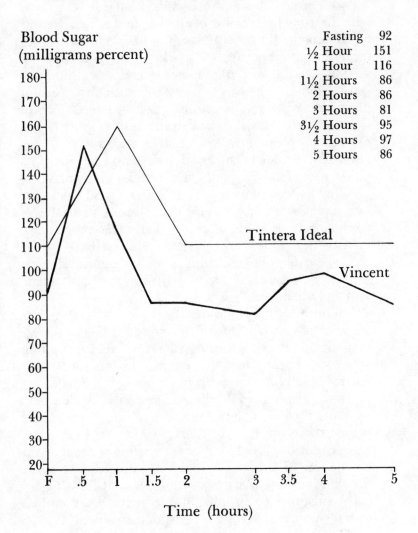

Blood Sugar
(milligrams percent)

Fasting	92
½ Hour	151
1 Hour	116
1½ Hours	86
2 Hours	86
3 Hours	81
3½ Hours	95
4 Hours	97
5 Hours	86

Tintera Ideal

Vincent

Time (hours)

I set Vincent's total carbohydrate intake at 175 grams, with the usual prohibition of all sugar and caffein. He was to eat protein six times a day (normal servings at three meals and small portions at snacks), a lot of organ foods, such as liver, thymus gland, brains, and in addition to a general vitamin, he was to take 2,000 milligrams each of niacin and vitamin C, four times a day. Such megadoses of vitamins have proved to be helpful to schizophrenics. A mineral supplement was to be taken once a day.

Vincent attended a state university and after one of its big October football games, a month later, his nervousness and hyperactivity returned. It was logical to suspect excitement over the game and a few slip-ups in his diet as dominant factors. He also reported an accompanying increase in fatigue. However, despite this setback, he did report general progress. At this point, two more B-vitamin supplements were added to his daily routine: pantothenic acid and vitamin B_6.

A month later, his mother phoned to say that he was better, but over the next few months his gains were periodically matched by losses. He would start going away from home. Once Vincent was missing for a week, during which time he had been smoking marijuana; one time he hospitalized himself voluntarily. At his next regular office visit, however, he had made remarkable strides: there was no "dust" in his brain, the tub water wasn't "cutting" him now, and he rarely worried about people watching him. Although he was left on basically the same routine, he was cautioned about limiting his daily consumption of milk to one quart, because of its carbohydrate and excessive phosphorus content.

Vincent's life was a continuing, unfinished book as he struggled into his twenties. For a while he was much more relaxed, and then his aggressiveness and insomnia returned. When he began refusing his diet, deterioration promptly set in. Vincent did not return for further checkups and I don't know what happened to him.

Vincent's case produced both pluses and minuses. He and his parents found that nutrition can be effective in serious behavioral disorders. His progress could be charted in direct proportion to how well he stayed on his diet. But the case also demonstrated that keeping the older teenager or young adult on a nutritional regimen can be a very trying task.

The main lesson that Vincent taught us is that no time should be wasted in putting a child on the carbohydrate control program and shoring up any metabolic flaws with supplements, while entirely cutting out sugar and caffein. Unfortunately, Vincent's parents didn't find this out when he was younger. But, in retrospect, we can see a number of revealing signs in his early childhood that may have presaged the malnutrition of affluence later on.

The most significant of these is that Vincent was a hyperactive child—the kind that, in the severe form, we call "the wild child."

If, as a young child, he had been treated, would he have become a schizophrenic a decade or so later? We cannot be certain of the answer. Some cases seem to defy every kind of known treatment. But any child will benefit from improved nutrition; for the vast majority, this alone will be a significant mood changer. The earlier a behavior problem is tackled, the more hopeful the outcome is likely to be. The most logical time to begin is when the child is a baby, if the early signs of a problem are recognized then. In some cases, for instance, the child may be afflicted with an environmental allergy which can be tested and thereafter avoided. Whatever the cause, years of unnecessary suffering may be prevented.

No longitudinal studies, based on significant numbers of patients over long periods of time, have been done on hyperactivity, but my own observations convince me there is a link between early hyperactivity and later behavioral disturbances. I have had numerous patients—late adolescents and young adults—who were severely disturbed emotionally, psychotic, or sociopathic, and in every case there was a history of hyperactivity in early childhood.

I do not mean that nutrition should be the only approach, but it should always be included. Some hyperkinetics may be latent schizophrenics. Others might later turn out to be neurotics, manic-depressives, or sociopaths. Early intervention through nutrition and, when needed, psychological counseling may prevent needless tragedy in later years.

What You Can Do

If you are the parent of a child with a behavior problem, there are a number of things you can do, nutritionally, that may get him to feel better and, at the same time, behave better. In infancy, feed him no commercial baby foods, sweets, or juices. In the preschool years, reward him with good food, not "goodies" and cold drinks. Limit treats to "high holidays" only—and never give caffein, whether it's in coffee, tea, pop, or chocolate.

Generally, the nutritional approach to hyperkinesis will also benefit other children, whether they have milder behavior problems or whether they are normal. In other words, the same program that can be helpful in treating hyperkinesis can be used to help prevent problems.

In the case of hyperkinesis, all possible organic causes for the unruly behavior should first be ruled out. A competent physician should check the child for faulty hearing, vision, or general health. Some children become hyperactive as a result of infections. In other instances, prescription drugs may bring on hyperactivity in certain sensitive children. When temper outbursts persist, a neurological examination may be wise.

Ideally, correction of your child's eating habits should be done in coöperation with your physician. If your doctor is not interested in exploring this approach, you may write to the Adrenal Metabolic Research Society of the Hypoglycemia Foundation (P.O. Box 98, Fleetwood, Mt. Vernon, New York 10052) or the International Association of Metabology (2236 Suree Ellen Lane, Altadena, California 91001) for a roster of physicians in your area who are interested in blood sugar and behavior.

If all else fails, and you wish to take matters into your own hands, you may do the following:

1. Get a carbohydrate gram counter as a guide and limit the child's daily carbohydrates to the following formula, according to age:

    2–6 years old, 75 grams

    6–10 years old, 115 grams

    10–15 years old, 135 grams

    Rapidly growing teenagers, 150–250 grams

2. Eliminate refined sugar as completely as possible, including syrups, honeys, and jellies.

3. Eliminate all caffein, whether it's in coffee, tea, colas (including those without "cola" in the name, such as *Dr. Pepper* and *Tab*), some root beer, or chocolate.

4. Restrict fruit and juice to breakfast only. Limit milk to one quart a day in a teenager, eighteen ounces for ten years and under.

5. Serve protein (meat, eggs, fish, or chicken) three times a day, seven days a week—lean cuts, when possible.

6. Use a simple digestive enzyme with meals, such as Viokase or Entozyme, if fatigue is a major problem. These usually can be purchased in the drug store without a prescription, although this may vary from state to state.

7. Give a balanced B–complex capsule twice a day. A

good guide is to see if has at least 5-10 milligrams of vitamin B_6 in it. Most other components of the B-complex are usually adequate if the B_6 (pyridoxine) is; some inadequate formulas measure B_6 in micrograms instead of milligrams. Read the labels! (*Sugarless* health food store liquid is recommended for children too young to swallow a tablet.)

    8. Administer daily additional doses of vitamin C:

        1–3 years old, 100 milligrams twice a day

        3–6 years old, 100 milligrams three times a day

        6–12 years old, 250 milligrams twice a day

        12 years old and up, 500 milligrams twice a day

    9. Give a complete mineral, vitamin, and trace element preparation, with care not to exceed 10,000 units of vitamin A and 800 units of vitamin D daily.

    10. Build the child up emotionally by attending to the psychological aspects while waiting for him to straighten out with nutrition. Go heavy on love, and light on punishment.

Once the child has been on a nutritional program for a month or more you will be in a better position to decide if he can benefit additionally by psychological counseling or supportive therapy. But improvement in his diet and physical condition is essential first, in order to obtain a realistic picture. Furthermore, until the child is built up nutritionally, no supportive therapy can be fully effective, for the child won't be able to listen attentively to the therapist.

ALTERNATIVE PROGRAM NO. 1 (LOW FAT, LOW CHOLESTEROL)

If the above ten step program does not achieve satisfactory results, some children have improved after limiting their fats and cholesterol intake. The following routine may prove helpful.

Follow the steps as listed in the original program, with the following modifications:

1. Low protein diet with lean meats, fish, poultry.
2. Restrict fats and oils.
3. Make up calories, as needed, with fibrous starchy foods such as potatoes, yams, cabbage, and other vegetables.

There are several reasons why the low fat and cholesterol diet may bring about better psychosomatic (body and mind) response in certain children.

1. It affords better blood sugar control.
2. It gives better control of appetite.
3. It reduces nervous disorders.
4. It promotes better attention and learning.
5. It gives better control of resistance to infection as a result of improved phagocytic action.

Other medical benefits of the low fat, low cholesterol diet (which also lowers the animal protein content in the diet) are that it:

1. Increases complex starches and fiber of all kinds, which lowers the cholesterol.
2. Decreases simple sugars which otherwise would elevate the triglycerides (another type of fat in the blood).
3. Increases intake of B-complex vitamins in grains.
4. Reduces the incidence of intestinal diseases, including colitis, constipation, and cancer.
5. Promotes better weight control.
6. Promotes better sleep habits.

ALTERNATIVE PROGRAM NO. 2 (ADDITIVES, SALICYLATES AVOIDANCE)

If results still do not occur, the following innovations can be made from the original program:

1. Restriction of all artificial coloring, flavoring agents, and additives. Processed foods, products, and

beverages containing these substances include ice cream, oleomargarine, luncheon meats, mint flavors, frankfurters, gum, jello, candies, Kool-Aid and similar beverages, all soft drinks, tea, and diet drinks.

2. Avoidance of salicylates (the active ingredient found in aspirin and many similar drugs) as prescribed in Dr. Ben F. Feingold's routine (presented in his book, *Why Your Child Is Hyperactive*), or as supervised by your physician.

3. Consult a doctor for medication if nutritional measures fail to control the hyperactivity.

ALTERNATIVE PROGRAM NO. 3 (NERVOUS DISORDERS OF A MAJOR DEGREE)

1. Continue with the original program, but discuss with an interested doctor the use of single vitamins B_3 (niacin), B_6, pantothenic acid, C, E, and inositol in large amounts.

2. Megavitamin programs should be monitored by a doctor once a month for signs of effects on a) nutritional status, b) liver enzyme levels, and c) urinary complaints.

ALTERNATIVE PROGRAM NO. 4 (METHODS OF CONTROLLING HYPERACTIVITY AND EMOTIONAL DISTURBANCES DUE TO ALLERGIES)

If other methods, including psychological counseling, do not produce normal behavior in the child, he could be sensitive to something he is exposed to in his food, water, air, clothing, or other parts of his environment. In cases where nothing else helps, one of the following approaches may be useful.

164

1. Conventional skin testing by an allergist may turn up an unexpected sensitivity to some substance.

2. The cytotoxic blood test, devised by Dr. William Bryan of St. Louis, may reveal a delayed allergic rection to foods.

3. A total environmental analysis—testing reactions to various components in the air (such as automobile exhaust, gas and paint fumes), the water that is consumed (for additives or pollutants), or food ingested (for undesirable chemicals or pollutants such as lead and mercury).

6

Why Some Children Don't Learn

Most of the time, when a child's behavior problem is solved, he begins to do better in school. In the case of the hyperactive child, the other children benefit as well, for the classroom can finally settle down to the lessons. However, on some occasions the child's learning problems may be more evident than behavior, even though they are linked like two pieces to the same puzzle; if one is improved, the other also improves.

There are other instances when the child exhibits a learning disability but is behaving properly. It is well to explore the reasons for lagging performance as soon as it is spotted.

A good beginning when you are concerned about your child's school record is to ask the teacher these three questions:

1. How much interest does he display in his work?
2. What does he accomplish?
3. How well does he get along with the other children?

166

A conference with the teacher, who sees your child in a different environment than that at home, may provide insights for both of you. The teacher may be aware of specific problems the child is facing in acquiring information, in reading, writing, or mathematics.

Learning disorders, unlike physical growth, do not involve "stages." Such problems refer specifically to children after the age of six, when they are in school. Developmental delay at an earlier age, when the child is learning to walk and talk, is a different ball game entirely.

If your child seems to be having definite problems in learning, your pediatrician should check the child for possible causes. Just as in behavior problems, specific medical problems may be at the heart of it. In fact, all of the factors that may bring on hyperactivity can also cause learning problems. The doctor can examine such factors as poor nutrition, eye function, and poor hearing. Any chronic nasal condition could be associated with mucous behind the ear drums, which affects hearing. Any visual dysperception or lack of coördination between hand and eye could show up in classroom performance. In some cases, the child may be consistently below par, which would certainly influence his enthusiasm about his work. A doctor's examination often will resolve a lot of worry.

Nine-year-old Willis's case provides some insight into the learning problems that affect many children today. Like most children who don't live up to scholastic expectations, Willis also had health and behavioral problems. He was hyperactive—not a "wild child," but too active to sit still. He constantly walked about the room, picking at his cuticles. In cool weather he had a hacking cough and constantly sniffed. For a year his nose had been stopped up.

Willis was making poor grades in school. His greatest difficulty was in reading. He had dyslexia, a special perceptual problem which meant he was unable to read more than a few lines with understanding, his eyes often transposing letters in a word as he read. The same difficulty seemed to carry over into his spelling. He had low grades in math. A slow worker, his work was usually inaccurate and his attention span short.

Unlike a lot of hyperactive children, however, Willis enjoyed good relations with his peers. He was very tender, considerate, and affectionate toward others. He had always played beautifully by himself as an infant and now he led others in games and creativity. He was good at football and loved to draw.

Based on previous experience, it seemed logical that if his health could be improved, his behavior would change. And if his overactivity could be helped, he would be able to settle down and learn.

At this point I reviewed his diet. The eggs he had for breakfast were overwhelmed by the cereal, jelly, and other refined carbohydrates he ate. His snacks usually were milk or colas in the mornings, ice cream in the afternoon. Desserts, sweet drinks, cookies, colas, and ice cream dominated his lunches. For seconds at dinner he took french fries and ice cream, again loading up on carbohydrates. His glucose tolerance curve is shown in Figure 6-1.

Willis began the Carbohydrate Control Program. His carbohydrates, at first, were restricted to 100 grams a day, including no more than 16 to 24 ounces of milk—two or three glasses. Gradually his limit was raised to 130 grams for a period of many months, keeping up with his changing needs as a growing boy. Like other children, he was given a general vitamin and digestive enzymes to make certain his body extracted all the nutrients from his food.

Within a month Willis was a changed boy. His nose

Figure 6-1. Willis' Glucose Tolerance Test

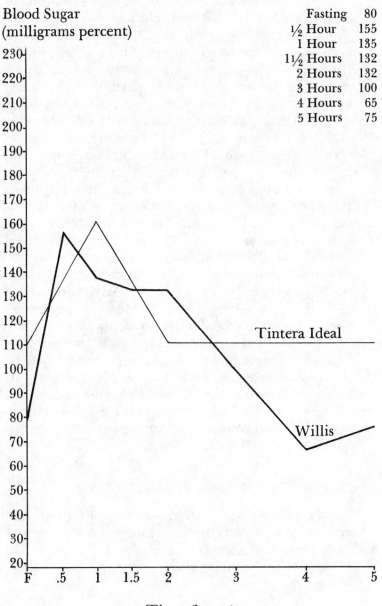

Blood Sugar
(milligrams percent)

Fasting	80
½ Hour	155
1 Hour	135
1½ Hours	132
2 Hours	132
3 Hours	100
4 Hours	65
5 Hours	75

Tintera Ideal

Willis

Time (hours)

remained "sniffy," but otherwise he was well physically. He was less restless and could sit still. Most significant of all, now he could do the multiplication tables.

Progress continued each time I saw him. After two months on the diet he still picked at his nails, but for the first time since infancy there was color in his face. He was less restless; his memory had improved. Willis remained on the diet and relished eating his high quality protein for meals and snacks as I had advised. After four months his mother said he was "a whole lot calmer" and his spelling was consistently better. He no longer paced the floor and did his work in school slowly, but accurately.

Problems of dyslexia are often improved by nutrition. In Willis's case he was reading at his grade level within a year after he had gone on this diet, his dyslexia had seemingly disappeared. Two years after his first office visit, he was "doing well academically."

Learning problems like Willis's, in varying degrees, are seen by parents and teachers every day. Many parents have the feeling that their sons or daughters are normal, yet they are failing in school or are not doing as well as they should. Although every child should be properly nourished, whether there is a learning problem or not, the poor performer especially should be eating soundly. In some cases that are severe or which do not respond readily, you should see your physician and the child's teacher to learn what kind of special training programs might be available in your locale.

Clues to Future Learning Problems

Dr. Mary S. Hoffman, medical director of Dallas Academy, a private school for children with learning disabilities, has compared the case histories of 100 children with learning problems to the cases of 200 students performing satisfactorily. From this study she formulated a screening test that could lead to early detection of learning problems.

If you have a child who is experiencing learning difficulties, you or your doctor may be able to use her findings in spotting a potential condition early. One isolated factor may not be significant, but several together may be clues to look out for. In many cases her findings may enable you to spot problems early enough to initiate a strong nutritional program that can help prevent the emergence of full-blown learning disorders.

Dr. Hoffman considered two factors:

1. The child's medical history before, during, and soon after birth.

   Prematurity
   Prolonged labor of the mother
   Difficult delivery
   Cyanosis due to a deficiency of oxygen in the blood
   Incompatibility of blood types
   Adoption

2. Developmental abnormalities.

   Late or abnormal creeping
   Late walking
   Prolonged tip-toe walking
   Late or abnormal speech
   Ambidexterity continuing after the age of seven

If the child's history contained one or two of these eleven characteristics, Dr. Hoffman classified the score as "suspicious"; if three, the case deserved more study; and if four or more, careful consideration would be mandatory. She emphasized that no single abnormality is indicative of a learning problem—a constellation of abnormalities would have to be present.

Scientific research has well documented the effects of

nutrition on learning. For example, Dr. Ruth F. Harrell and associates, studying thousands of women, compared the intelligence of offspring of women given vitamins during pregnancy and lactation. The population, in urban Norfolk, Virginia, was divided into four groups: the first, in which vitamin C tablets were added to the diet; the second, in which thiamine only was added; a third, in which thiamine, riboflavin, niacinamid, and iron supplemented the diet; and the fourth, in which only an inert placebo was used.

Intelligence of the women's offspring was measured at ages three and four. The results were striking. The mean intelligence of those children whose mothers had received vitamin supplements was "significantly higher" than those whose mothers had taken a placebo. Specifically, the more the variety of supplemental vitamins, the higher the intelligence of the children. Those with the highest average IQ were those whose mothers had taken the mixed vitaimins (thiamine, riboflavin, vitamin C, and iron). The ones whose mothers had taken only thiamine or vitamin C trailed behind those with the multivitamin supplementation. The placebo group was at the bottom in average intelligence scores.

Vitamin supplementation probably influenced the development of the central nervous system, which continues for the first two years of a child's life, and this probably made the difference in the intelligence scores. This double-blind study, reported in the medical journal *Metabolism,* has special relevance to the malnutrition of affluence, in which the child is very frequently deficient in sufficient quantities of vitamin C or the various factors in the B-complex.

Brain development is closely related to nutrition. The human brain's growth is essentially complete by the time the child is two years old. Poorly nourished children have been found not only to have smaller head sizes, on the average, but their brains also weighed less than those of the better-nourished children. In Chile, infants dying of malnutrition were found to have fewer brain cells than did children the same age dying from accidents.

As far back as 1929 researchers at the University of Chicago ran experiments on rats' learning ability when depleted of the B-complex vitamins. The test rats were depleted during their nursing period by the simple method of denying yeast and wheat germ from the diets of the nursing mother rats. In the control group, no such restrictions were made. After the nursing period, both groups were given adequate diets. The two groups of rats were then tested as to their maze-learning abilities. The comparisons were conclusive: the rats whose diets had been deficient in the B-complex during nursing were far below the normal rats in maze learning. "Normal rats are about twice as efficient as the depleted animals," noted researchers Siegfried Maurer and Loh Seng Tsai. A particularly telling observation was that "only one of the thirty-six B-deficient animals had achieved the median score of the control group." The study also discounted the possibility of genetic factors as having made the difference. Litters from the same parents were compared. "In every instance," the researchers observed, "the B-deficient litter exhibits a poorer record in maze learning than the control litter from the same parents."

Although the vitamins of the B-complex are highly important to learning, protein is also crucial. Dr. Herbert G. Birch and Joan Dye Gussow, citing research findings of others, have pointed out that low protein diets have caused deranged carbohydrate metabolism and changes in the endocrine system, and that protein-deprived experimental pigs had smaller brains than those fed protein. Of particular significance to the malnutrition of affluence is

173

one experiment cited, in which brain waves of the protein-deprived animals indicated abnormal brain functioning—*"especially among those on low-protein diets with added carbohydrate."* By decreasing the protein intake in experimental pigs, severe abnormalities were shown in both brain waves and brain structure. Researchers observed that on a rehabilitative diet outward signs of improvement frequently occurred first, followed by the brain waves' returning to normal. The last area to recover was the central nervous system.

A further insight into this problem is offered by Dr. Leonard Kryston, professor of endocrinology and metabology at Hahnemann Medical College, who consistently found an abnormal insulin secretion in children with learning disabilities. Insulin directly regulates blood sugar; thus, abnormal insulin secretion will result in an abnormal blood sugar. This leads to an abnormality of glucose to the brain and disturbs brain functions at all levels.

The volume of research over the past several decades should be sufficient to establish the importance of diet. To quote Drs. Emanuel Cheraskin and W. Marshall Ringsdorf, Jr., "The evidence suggests that *malnutrition* because of poor food choices is very likely a bigger problem than undernutrition."

At least one statistical study has shown the effectiveness of improved nutrition on learning behavior. Nancy Bower and Earl L. McCallon, conducting an appraisal of nutritional counseling in the Arlington, Texas, schools, concluded that a program, parallel to the one outlined in this book, led to a significant improvement of attention in class. Seventeen children were selected from among four schools on the basis of their lessened attention spans and were matched with control groups. The experimental groups showed a five-point increase from 18 to 23 on a scale of 30—a significant 28 percent rise—after nutritional intervention, while the control group rose from 23 to 24—a 4 percent increase.

Some children within the experimental group improved considerably more than others, and these were the ones who ate a high protein-low carbohydrate diet. Thus motivation probably linked to the parents' degree of interest in the program, appears to have been one factor. It provides a hint of what can be done.

"Caffeinism"—A Common Affliction

Throughout this book I have mentioned the deleterious effects of caffein upon children almost in the same breath as refined carbohydrates. But because "caffeinism" is so prevalent among school age children today, this subject deserves our special, detailed attention.

The effect of caffein consumption is difficult to separate from that of sugar and other refined carbohydrates. Usually the child who is consuming an overload of carbohydrates is also consuming caffeinated drinks. In many cases, neither he nor his parents will be aware of the amount of caffein that is being taken in.

Caffein is so commonly consumed today by everyone that we have forgotten that it is a drug. In earlier years it was used by doctors as a heart and respiratory stimulant during emergency conditions. Eventually, however, better treatment methods were developed and caffein was discontinued. Ironically, today it has come to be one of the most commonly-used drugs in this country, dispensed in business offices, in school corridors through soft-drink machines, and even at church socials. Preschoolers through elderly retirees faithfully get their daily "fixes."

In my own practice I have observed a definite relationship between behavior problems and caffeinism, which eventually shows up in school performances. For this reason I have saved this detailed discussion for this chapter, as the school age child or teenager is especially susceptible to this modern-day drug affliction.

What is the effect of caffein upon the body? First, it excites all levels of the central nervous system—the cortex (thinking level), the medulla (automation centers), and the spinal cord (distribution pathways). In moderate doses, caffein enhances functions, but in unpredictable ways. A moderate dose might range from 150 to 250 milligrams, the equivalent of two cups of coffee, three cups of tea, or three 12-ounce bottles of cola. Children are more susceptible to the drug than adults, because of their immature bodies and smaller masses. Furthermore, the effect may vary from one person to the next.

Unfortunately, in most caffeinated drinks there is also sugar. Many persons consume diet drinks without realizing that they may have caffein. Let us take a look at some of the popular soft drinks, for a more specific idea of their sugar and caffein contents.

Drink (10 oz)	Sugar Percent	Grams of Sugar	Equivalent in Tsps.	Milligrams of Caffein	Approx. Equivalent
Dr. Pepper	7–10	30	6	60	½ cup coffee
Diet Dr. Pepper	0	0	0	42	⅓ cup coffee
Coca Cola	11	33	6	54	½ cup coffee
Tab	0	0	0	36	¼ cup coffee
Mr. Pibb	11.5	33	6	0	0
Grape Drink	12	36	6	0	0
Orange Drink	12	36	6	0	0

One tends to think of caffein as "perking us up." It does, but then it lets us down. Many people feel the pick-up for one or two hours. Caffein is a biphasic drug. After the initial intake, auditory perception and hand–eye coordination are significantly impaired. These conditions are accompanied by mental confusion and poor concentration and only add to those problems the hyperactive-learning disabled child is already struggling with. In sensitive persons caffein may cause insomnia, restlessness, excitement, tense muscles, and tremulousness. These are also symptoms that are present in hyperactive children with learning problems; obviously the addition of caffein to the diet is going to add to the difficulty.

There are also certain ways in which caffein actively and directly interferes with the learning process. It may adversely affect a recently acquired motor skill in a task involving delicate muscular coordination and accurate timing. Tests have shown student performance to be worse in problems involving tactile discrimination and acoustic associations, two hours after moderate doses of caffein.

Not only does caffein tamper with the steady flow of blood sugar to the brain, but the side effects of that result may be expressed in a number of unexpected ways—nervousness, fatigue, and anxiety may increase.

Dr. John F. Greden, director of psychiatric research at the Walter Reed Medical Center, presented his observations on caffeinism at the 1974 annual meeting of the American Psychiatric Association. It is worth noting that Greden's list of symptoms coincide with those I have found in my own patients who have a history of consuming sugar and caffein.

177

CAFFEIN SYMPTOMS OBSERVED BY GREDEN

1. Nervousness, irritability
2. Tremulousness and muscle twitching.
3. Insomnia.
4. Sensory disturbance.
5. Autonomic nervous system instability with overbreathing, palpitations, flushing, and arrhythmias.
6. Diuresis (frequent urination).
7. Gastrointestinal troubles.
8. Headaches.
9. Patients do not respond to psychopharmacologic agents or nighttime hypnotics.
10. Children overactive or hyperkinetic.

COMPLAINTS OF CHILDREN ADDICTED TO CAFFEIN AND SUGAR

1. Hostility, rages, temper outbursts, and hyperactivity all prevalent.
2. Jerking, twitching, and awkwardness.
3. Most children exhibited irregular sleep habits.
4. Extreme skin sensitivity common.
5. Sighing, skipped heart beats, skin usually putty-gray or ashen in color.
6. Prolonged bedwetting common.
7. Virtually all children with hyper-impulse disorders drink caffein have stomach complaints.
8. Common symptom.
9. One-third experience no benefit on any drugs (including Ritalin) and one-third are worse.
10. Overactivity.

Everyone, including children, realizes that there is an ingredient in coffee "that keeps you awake." Some recognize that the same thing is in tea, a few understand it to be in Coca Cola. But most people appear to be astounded to learn that caffein is in many diet colas such as Diet Pepsi, Diet Shasta Cola, and Diet Dr. Pepper. Chocolate itself contains 20 milligrams of caffein per ounce. Since elimination of caffein is as important as avoidance of sugar for the child with learning or behavior problems, it is important to carefully study everything that the child takes into his body. The best rule of thumb to follow is, as I have mentioned earlier, to avoid all "brown" drinks, which would include coffee, tea, colas (whether advertised as a cola or not), and chocolate. An exception to this rule would be carob, which is "brown" but does not contain caffein and is used by many families instead of chocolate. It can be obtained in most health food stores.

School Behavior and Nutrition

If we accept the evidence of newspaper accounts, teachers' observations, and parents' comments, disturbing behavior is one of the most troublesome challenges facing schools today. All sorts of explanations have been given for it, and as many solutions offered. But the problem seems only to be spreading. Children are spanked and placed in "quiet rooms" in order to control their rebelliousness and behavioral outbursts. This often seems to lead to confrontations between parents and school officials.

Many teachers are quitting or are getting out of the classrooms by going into other facets of education, such as counseling. One teacher who gave in to retirement after twenty-five years in the classrooms emphasized, in a letter

179

to a syndicated columnist, that she had turned in her chalk and gradebook strictly because of the children's behavior. "I daresay there is not a teacher in America who would not agree how much students have changed in just the last five years," she wrote. "This past year, I have seen children defy teachers openly and loudly with the most obscene of the obscenities; with taunts and their own cruel kind of put-downs; and with personal, physical assaults. Typewriters, laboratory equipment, whatever not nailed down has been stolen; schools vandalized; records destroyed."

This, she hastened to say, had not occurred in the urban slums but in rural middle-America, and she noted a shocking trend: "I have watched the ranks of the 'good kids' shrink from a 90 percent majority to the present approximately 30 percent."

We would not attempt to lay all of the blame on the malnutrition of affluence, but a great deal of the fault must be placed there. If such things could be measured and compared, we believe very strongly that a significant relationship would be revealed between the deteriorating American diet and the deteriorating behavior of its young. For one thing, shouting obscenities around parents have been constant findings in my patients; strangely, they are one of the earliest signs of improvement after carbohydrate control and caffein elimination. My own observations indicate such obscene language is related to nervousness, which is any maladjustment of the nervous system.

It is especially important that both the home and the school coördinate to offer the best nutrition available for school age children. School meals, whether in the cafeteria or the lunch box, should contain proper foods, include some protein at each meal, and care should be taken that they are free of sugar and caffein. Unfortunately, some school lunches and breakfasts are loaded with sugar in the form of sweet rolls, doughnuts, desserts, and juices, and contain no protein. A simple snack containing nothing but whole grain bread, butter, and milk would be better, for at least it would provide B-complex in the bread, protein in the milk along with available carbohydrates and fat.

In order to do all it can to exclude sugar and caffein from children's diets, a school's administration would have to remove soft drink and candy machines from the school property. This might be a courageous move that many school administrators would hesitate to carry out. Often school activities are partially funded from the income of these machines. However, when parents, teachers, and children all understand how the products of these machines may play a significant role in disrupting the learning process, cooperation may result. The key may be judicious and diplomatic conferences between teachers, administrators, and parents or PTA groups. One junior high teacher in the Dallas Public Schools has observed the benefits of such a change.

"Last year," he said, "the Coca-Cola Bottling Company removed all their machines for about two weeks. The behavior of the students was markedly changed for the better during the absence of the cold drinks."

My own medical experience in treating children with learning and behavior difficulties confirms his conclusion. A coördinated effort of both the school and home could bring about improvements in our children's nutrition of which we would all be proud.

7

Making Household Pediatrics Work

The success of any medical or nutritional program depends on the coöperation of the patient. In pediatrics, this means the patient and *both* of his parents by:

1. Insuring that the child adheres to his nutritional regimen.

2. Maintaining an adequate supply of the proper nutrients, especially protein. This may prove to be a somewhat complicated assignment, since we face the realities of a crippled economy and high protein foods are usually expensive.

Both factors are essential if the carbohydrate control program is to work. The success of family after family in getting their children to "eat right" is proof enough that others can do the same. But the most realistic step, and the most helpful one, is for the parents to adopt the program for themselves, too. It will help their health, as well as that of their children.

Armed with the knowledge that is in this book and consciously striving to steer the child in the right direction, parents soon will find that there is quite a lot they can do, merely by changing their child's food and drink patterns. These successes should be encouragement enough to insure a conscientious follow-up on the program.

Nothing is more basic and crucial to good health than a child's eating habits. Yet, some parents will say "I feel sorry for her," implying that taking their child off sweets and caffein is too great a burden to impose upon one of such tender years. Which is more important, to feel sorry for the child when these substances will continue to affect learning, health, and behavior or to help the child get well and remain healthy?

Dietary changes should be firmly implemented, but never in a harsh manner. In instances where you are dealing with teenagers or are trying to change the entire family's food habits, it is usually best to modify the diet slowly, in order not to be discouraging or seem too authoritarian. You must allow time for withdrawal symptoms to subside in the caffeinated drink addicts: headaches, nausea, nervousness, and fatigue. The "cold turkey" approach is not recommended. Gradual withdrawal will create less strain and will make life easier for all concerned. You don't have to worry about success at all the first week, for this will be a period of transition as you keep count of carbohydrate grams and become more aware of the suspicious foods. Once these are firmly in mind, it is time to start revamping the diet—bringing in the protein, vegetables, fruits, and whole grain cereals and breads, while gradually phasing out the sugars and refined carbohydrates. It may help to remember that good food will help change the child's attitudes. After a while he will lose his taste for bad food.

183

The best approach at home is to improve the entire family's diet. The same sweets and caffeinated drinks that damage young lives are not any more helpful to other members of the family. If desserts and cola drinks are always on the table, but are forbidden to one child, it should not be surprising if he becomes resentful. Offering valuable resistance foods to everyone will be much fairer. They all can then make their selection from high value foods only.

In instances where the sugar addict is extraordinarily hooked on the sweet taste, the pressure may be relieved during a transition period by substituting liquid saccharine in cereals and homemade drinks. Instead of sugar, recipes may substitute white carob syrup, liquid saccharine, or tupelo honey, which may be purchased from health food stores. A good guide for such recipes is *Sugarless Cookery for the Gourmet* by Elsie Maye Peckham.

There is at present a controversy over saccharine, which you should take into consideration. Very high levels of saccharine and cyclamates have been shown in laboratory experiments to produce cancer in rats. It would be highly unusual for the human to take in, proportionally, the amount used in the experiments. For example, the Mead Johnson company, which manufactures baby food and vitamins, ran the research figures through their computer to check them against the quantity of cyclamates then used in their chewable vitamin tablet. The result was that a child would have to take 5,000 vitamin tablets a day for the rest of his life if he were to ingest as much of the artificial sweetener as the test animals were given. For this reason, many researchers and doctors have questioned the validity of the evidence. Ideally, it would be best to avoid both sugar and its artificial substitutes. But in severe cases you might find these substitutes helpful during "easing off" periods. There is no doubt about sugar's harmful effects.

It may be helpful to review some tips for phasing out a craving for sweets in your child.

1. Do not create negativism by scolding, threatening, or making excessive demands.

2. From time to time make sweet-tasting substitutes available, by consulting a good cookbook designed for those with low blood sugar or by occasionally purchasing candy bars, made of fructose alone which are sold in health food stores (if frequent infections are not a problem).

3. If (2) doesn't work, assess the state of rebellion in the child and, based on your judgment, allow the child to "blow it" once a month.

4. Teach little children how to manage themselves at birthday parties. Offer some nutritional advice to the parent in charge.

5. Attempt nutritional rehabilitation for the entire family, to the point of sacrifice, if necessary, and keep harmful items out of the house.

6. Win the father's and grandparents' interest by explanations whenever necessary.

7. Look behind the scenes for psychological causes of rebellion and find a psychologist to work with the child.

8. Draw the child's glucose tolerance test graph, discuss the problem in his terms, and end with a cheerful note.

By the time the child is about three, the nutrition-minded parents encounter a major frustration: the birthday party. They can substitute milk or a carob-milk drink for the colas and chocolates, fruit nibbles instead of candy, and, if the season is right, watermelon can be served. If a cake is necessary on this one day of the year, they should insure that it is made of whole wheat or soy flour and sweetened as lightly as possible with tupelo honey.

If the child is invited to another child's party, it is a different matter. If the hostess-mother is a friend, she might be persuaded to offer substitutes for the risky foods—always tactfully. As a last resort, you can encourage the child to eat sparingly of the birthday cake. The results will depend on the age of the child, how well directed he is, and his overall condition of health.

It is extremely important that the child get off to as sound a start as possible, as early in life as possible, in his nutrition. The older the child, the more difficult it is to turn him around from his sugar and caffein addictions.

Early discipline and parental guidance are particularly important. The anti-health factors seem to be pervasive and are often subtle. During an hour long double feature in which thirty minutes of "Peanuts" were followed by thirty minutes of Dr. Seuss, the major sponsors were a sweet cola drink, doughnuts, a breakfast cereal, and a chocolate product. Certainly children should not be deprived of these popular programs, but the parents can seek means to blunt the impact of the commercials; giving healthful snacks is one way.

Parents should watch TV with their children and point out the offensive nature of commercials when appropriate. If they take the time to analyze these food commercials, and show how they emphasize the wrong foods, the child can then begin a conscious examination of what is going on. Maybe after a while he will become knowledgeable enough to help his friends.

As the child approaches the age of six and starts to go to school, it becomes more difficult to insure that he is getting proper nutrition. But it can be done, and it is worth every bit of effort. If the child is bright and cooperative, almost any tactful, child-oriented approach will probably work.

The School-Age Child

Two approaches may be taken for the school-age child. He may take his lunch, which is the surest way, for then the parent is responsible. If well done and wrapped in wax paper, meat will keep several hours and can be used with whole grain bread in a sandwich. Protein powder can be mixed in with milk in a thermos or protein tablets can be given to the child. If the child eats in the school cafeteria, the problem is more complex, for he must be educated to know what to take and what to avoid. Desserts and vending machines may overwhelm the carboholic and caffein addict. However, the child can be taught to shun all desserts and any other dishes that seem to be sugared. For a drink, he can stick to plain milk or buttermilk. If he likes chocolate milk, you can give him milk mixed with carob powder when he gets home, or in his thermos. Carob looks like chocolate and tastes better but contains no caffein. By selecting protein foods like meat, fish, eggs, and cheese, the child may be able to come through the cafeteria line in good shape. If he can be instructed gradually and patiently in which foods to take and which to avoid, it would also contribute to the development of self-discipline. By becoming responsible for his actions at the lunch table it is likely he will become responsible in other ways, as well.

If parents are willing to invest the time and energy, quite a lot can be done about the child's eating environment at school. Cafeterias can save a great deal of money by cutting out sugar-laden desserts entirely.

Improvement of school lunches and eradication of cold drink and candy machines from the schools can be brought about. If there is a large number of people interested at the grass roots level, changes can be made. By

187

informing yourselves and seeing that your friends are made aware, you will have made a great beginning. Then you will be in a better position to assess the school's food program and vending machine situation. Most supporters of the vending machines point out they are a source of money with which "specials" for the school are brought. When it is recognized that these extras come at the expense of the children's health, many people will be willing to find other ways of raising money. For instance, cheese, milk, nuts, fruits, and juices may also be dispensed in vending machines.

The renovation of an entire school's food program could be one of the most rewarding events in a community's life. It can be accomplished when there is a dedicated group of parents who are willing to put forth the time and effort that will be necessary. Mrs. Ann Moran, mother of one of my patients, has become an expert on this subject. Based upon her study of the problem and her recommendations I can suggest the following courses of action:

1. Change the contents of the vending machines through the PTA's influence upon the school board and the vending machine companies.

2. Prevail upon the school board to incorporate nutrition lectures into the curriculum.

3. Organize mothers' clubs for those whose children are affected by sugar, caffein, and additives such as the "Feingold substances."

4. Have PTA representatives attend leading food conferences where experts are now presenting research to show how diet affects behavior.

5. Try to find a nutrition oriented doctor as an ally who also will talk to medical school faculties and county medical societies about the problem.

In beginning the carbohydrate control program at

home, it is of utmost importance to secure the good will of the child. This should be the first step in changing the child's eating habits. There is little point in discussing it with the child until he's in a frame of mind that is receptive. Find something to build the child up with, before showing him what's wrong. If he has been nice to someone, tell him. "You did a good job there." A parent should never hesitate to show appreciation to the child.

A number of tips may prove helpful to the parent who is embarking on a new nutritional course. "Don't stuff like a goose," is a good rule. If a child has suffered fatigue between meals, a light snack may be helpful in tiding him over to the next meal. But in cases where the child eats six times a day—three meals and three snacks—there is still no reason for him to overeat.

He should eat just enough between meals to keep the blood sugar level up. This might consist of a snack of a slice of cheese or a spoonful of tuna fish on a wedge of whole-grain bread or several nuts. Frequent eating of moderate portions of proper food will not add to the child's weight. Studies at Northwestern University have shown that one large meal adds weight, while the same amount of food in six feedings doesn't.

Along with this there is another rule: never eat fruit by itself. Fruit, fruit juice, honey, and orange juice, for instance, contain fructose, glucose, and sucrose, all simple sugars. Children who are particularly sensitive and nervous may be made more nervous by eating a banana by itself, for example. But fruit eaten with protein food is an excellent selection, as the protein supplies a stable blood sugar level and acts to "buffer" the faster-absorbing sugars from the fruit.

I have seen mothers break down into tears as they explained how difficult it had been for them to change their children's diets. But the key is to arm yourself with a

189

knowledge of foods and to initiate changes as gradually and in as relaxed a manner as possible.

There are any number of ways in which a child can easily be fed a high protein meal. Egg, meat, or fish can be cooked in different styles. Cheese can be used in cooking. You can put at least one egg in a batch of soy flour pancake batter. Jane Kinderlehrer's delightful book, *Confessions of a Sneaky Organic Cook*, provides a number of examples.

A little ingenuity will often solve some of your problems. For instance, although most of the packaged breakfast foods/cereals sold today are heavily sugared, you can make your own. Here is what one mother did, by combining a series of health-promoting items.

FRAN'S SUGAR-FREE CEREAL

Ingredients

Rolled oats	Raisins
Sunflower seeds	Brazil nuts
Sesame seeds	Walnuts
Wheat-germ	Carob powder (if desired)
Bran	

Directions: Use each ingredient in the proportion to which its taste appeals to you and your child, with care not to overbalance the raisins, which have a lot of natural sugar, nor the nuts, which are high in fats. First, bake the oats in a pan for 20 to 30 minutes at 350°F degrees, to make them more digestible. Then mix all the ingredients together thoroughly in any desired quantity. A large mixing bowl will make enough to last for a week or more at a time. One of the nuts or seeds may be omitted, if desired. Served with milk, this cereal is a nutritious, concentrated food.

At times, the parent can use the child's regular eating

habits as a guide for changing them. It does not matter what a child eats at a particular meal, as long as the essential nutrients are included and none of the risky foods is available. For instance, if a child likes hamburger, then there's nothing wrong with his having a home-cooked hamburger (without the white buns) for breakfast. Some children may not like eggs for breakfast but will eat them at another meal.

Above all, one thing should be kept in mind. Changing a child's diet is an art. You learn by doing. As you gain more experience and keep working at it with an eye toward improving your techniques and knowledge, the more artistic you are likely to become in your endeavor. If you meet disappointments, don't give up. Good results sometimes take months.

Despite its crucial importance, however, food cannot do everything. There are a certain number of children who seem to defy all attempts at improvement. Serious medical problems could be the reason and the child should be taken to a qualified physician.

Economy Tips

Assuming that your child cooperates and helps make the carbohydrate control program a success, there is another problem that must be solved. How do you insure that he has an adequate source of proper nutrition, particularly when protein is so expensive?

A complaint that is sometimes expressed by mothers is, "But meats and other protein dishes cost so much!" Yet when they got into the mechanics of actually putting the high protein food on the table, they found that, over all, the cost was not high. For one thing, they were no longer spending money on "starvation" foods. An analysis, by weight and cost, of foods such as soda pop, potato chips, cookies, pizzas, cakes, and pies, is usually enough to convince the homemaker that these are expensive foods.

A sample list of junk and healthful foods, with comparative prices, will illustrate this point. Although prices may change from one month to the next, this roster should provide an indication of how one food stacks up with the other in terms of price and quality.

JUNK FOODS		GOOD FOODS	
Soft drinks:		Milk, ½ gallon	$ .79
Coke, three 32 oz.			
bottles,	$1.00		
Dr. Pepper, 6 cans,	1.32	Whole-wheat bread,	
Potato chips, 8 oz. bag	.77	1 lb. loaf	.79
Ice cream sundae cups		Yogurt, plain,	
package of a dozen		four 8 oz. boxes	1.00
3 oz. cups	1.49	Cheese, mild chedder, 10 oz.	1.19
Jelly, blackberry, 18 oz. jar	.99	Whole-wheat wafers, 7¼ oz.	.59
Cheese-flavored crackers,		Cracked wheat, 24 oz.	.75
16 oz.	.69	Tabouly (Bulgar wheat,	
Enchilada dip,		dehydrated vegetables)	
10½ oz. can	.59	salad mix or	
		dip dry	
Kellog's Sugar Smacks, 18 oz.	1.03	mix, 8 oz.	.95
		Granola, 16 oz.	1.39
		Familia (without honey),	
		12 oz.	1.19

In all cases, the "good" foods greatly surpass the "junk" foods in quality. In some of the comparisons, good food is cheaper than junk food, ounce for ounce; sometimes junk food is cheaper by weight. But what is important to remember is that we don't need to eat as much nutritious food as we do the easily-absorbed junk foods that leave us hungry and wanting more. Because of this fact, even when good food costs more, it will go farther and leave our bodies more satisfied and in better shape. When we compare the above items on the basis of nutritional value, the good foods easily win.

One thing should be remembered: if you don't spend money for high quality food, you'll spend more money on drugs and doctors' bills later.

With that in mind, three essential steps might be considered in order to economize on food in this era of rising food prices:

1. Take the money that is normally spent on junk foods and spend it on high quality food, insuring that there is sufficient protein.

2. Combine vegetable protein foods with animal proteins, in order to enhance and extend the animal protein foods. There are infinite possibilities here, such as beans with stew meat or carrots and other vegetables in a casserole or meatloaf.

3. Use the often overlooked, but very valuable, organ meats such as sweetbreads (thymus gland or pancreas), brains, calf's liver, heart, and tongue. In addition to being bargains, they are easily digested and are high in minerals and the B vitamins. In fact, they are excellent food for anyone. Tripe should also be included in meals.

Here are some sample menus. A good policy to follow is to use just one animal protein food at a meal. This will help reduce the fat intake.

BREAKFAST

Small glass of fruit juice or whole fruit
An egg (or ham or sausage that is not preserved with sodium nitrite or sodium nitrate)
A slice of whole-grain bread (butter optional)
A glass of milk
Wheat germ, or cooked whole grain cereal

193

LUNCH

Meat, poultry, or fish
Salad
Vegetables
One slide of whole grain bread (butter optional)
Milk
If the child is taking his lunch to school:
Best choice—A sandwich of chicken salad, roast beef, or tuna
fish
Second choice—A peanut butter sandwich, with the natural
unhydrogenated, unsweetened type of peanut butter

DINNER

Soup
Vegetables
Meat, fish, or poultry
One slice of whole grain bread (butter optional)
Fruit or cheese for dessert
Milk

Snacks, if given at mid-morning, mid-afternoon, or at bedtime, should be chosen from meat, eggs, cheese, fish, nuts, natural peanut butter, or vegetables.

Food supplements, such as protein powder, are usually all right if they contain no sugar, but they should never be used as substitutes. Don't ever discount the value of food! It's the raw material from which we manufacture our energy.

For those who wish to explore ways in which to economize while delivering a high protein diet to the family table, the U.S. Department of Agriculture has prepared two home and garden bulletins, "Money-Saving Main Dishes" (No. 43; 55 cents) and "Your Money's Worth in Foods" (No. 183; 50 cents), both of which are available from the *U.S. Government Printing Office*, Washington D.C. 20402. The former is filled with recipes, while the latter covers shopping tips. An excellent guide is *Nutrition—Applied Personally*, published by the International College of Applied Nutrition, Box 386, La Habra, California 90631.

Among the better buys of good quality protein are whole chickens and frozen fish. Perch, cod, and whiting are usually good buys all year round, and canned fish like pink light salmon, tuna, sardines, mackerel, and herring should not be overlooked. Cottage cheese is also a good source of protein and can be used in cooking certain dishes, such as lasagna with whole grain noodles. (I do not consider cottage cheese a complete protein source, however, since it is a milk product.) Leftover meats should be used in casseroles, salads, or sandwiches; the bones can be cooked with beans or soup.

Buying Tips

Several precautions should be taken during the buying process. Careful label reading should always be a part of every shopping experience. All ingredients should be carefully scrutinized for additives and any hint of sugar that may have been added in various forms. As I have mentioned, even on baby foods and juices, labels sometime note, "sugar added to achieve balance of sweetness" or "sugar added to enhance natural sweetness." This is creating an addiction almost before the infant has his eyes open; it should not be tolerated in food for any age group. Sometimes sugar is disguised on the label, and parades under its various technical names such as sucrose and fructose. Dextrose and corn syrup are equally undesirable simple sugars. Other sweeteners such as sorbitol and mannitol should also be avoided. Even natural fruit juices sometimes have sugar added; reading the label on the container is the only way to tell.

The best beginning rule on drinks is to avoid all dark brown ones, as I have emphasized. This takes care of caffeinated drinks from colas to chocolate and even those that we do not normally think of as caffein-laden drinks. All carbonated or any artificially made concoctions should also be avoided.

One of the most dangerous ingredients to look for on labels is sodium nitrite. Sodium nitrite is commonly found in meat products like bacon and frankfurters, as well as other processed foods. It is now the most controversial food additive since cyclamates. In a baby, a high dose of sodium nitrite can cause methemoglobinemia, a disorder affecting the hemoglobin in blood which can be fatal. But that is just a beginning. Nitrites are now linked with cancer. According to Dr. Michael F. Jacobson of the Center for Science in the Public Interest, Washington, D.C., "the worst offender and probably the most dangerous food in the supermarket is bacon." Until the government moves against nitrites, he adds, "your best bet is to stay away from the hot dog stand and *don't bring home the bacon.*" As for the commercial hot dog, aside from its nitrite content, Jacobson emphasized that it "has decayed to the point where it has only two more grams of protein than the fluffy white coffin in which it is encased." His advice to those who like hot dogs and sausages is to buy nitrite-free products from health food stores and certain supermarkets that stock them. Bratwurst and breakfast sausages, he notes, do not contain nitrite, since the industry relies upon refrigeration to preserve them.

A thorough knowledge of foods must be a continuing form of education in our lives. It is essential to our health and each day it is becoming more of an economic necessity. Although most of us know the pitfalls of packaged ready-to-eat cereals, many still do not know that, dollar for dollar, oatmeal provides more protein than any other grain food product. And today, more than ever before, we need to know that we can stretch certain dishes by adding skim milk powder, soybean flour, or brewer's yeast to ground meat. By using these items instead of potatoes and bread crumbs, the cook increases the protein value of the meal. By remembering that high-grade proteins team up with the less complete proteins, we can combine food substances in order to enhance the value of all of them.

If we are to make it all work, by seeing that our families eat what we put before them, we should remember the friendly hint offered by the International College of Applied Nutrition: "The more you can do without pointing it out in the family, the better. Be subtle. Enlist their aid. Quiet discussions apart from mealtime are better than mealtime confrontations." The goal, after all, of our nutritional program is health and happiness. One is unthinkable without the other, and it seems reasonable to believe that no child is going to be happy unless he is first healthy.

A Note On Sources

The reader who wishes to pursue some of the topics discussed herein further may find the following sources useful. They also will provide references to some of the material upon which the various chapters were based.

1. Mood-Changing Foods

Charts of Tintera's "ideal standard" are show in John W. Tintera, *Hypoadrenocorticism* (Scarsdale, N.Y.: The Hypoglycemia Foundation, 1966), pp. 43 *et seq*. This booklet is mainly a collection of Dr. Tintera's technical articles published in various medical journals.

The three groups of blood sugar curves were first presented in Hugh W.S. Powers, Jr., "Dietary Measures to Improve Behavior and Achievement" *Academic Therapy* IX, 3; (Winter, 1973-74), pp. 203–14, which is largely based upon an earlier paper given before the Texas Association for Children With Learning Disabilities, Austin, Oct. 16, 1970.

The concept of orthomolecular medicine is in Linus Pauling, "Orthomolecular Psychiatry," *Science* (vol. 160; April 19, 1968), 265-71, and Linus C. Pauling, "The New Medicine?" *Nutrition Today* (September/October, 1972), pp. 18-23.

2. *Fuel for Human Machinery*

A variety of materials proved helpful for this chapter. The differences among persons are explored in Roger J. Williams, *Biochemical Individuality: The Basis for the Genetotrophic Concept* (New York: John Wiley and Sons, 1956; Austin, The University of Texas Press). A popular version is Roger J. Williams, *You Are Extraordinary* (New York: Random House, 1968; paperback, Pyramid Books, 1971).

Herbert G. Birch and Joan Dye Gussow, *Disadvantaged Children: Health, Nutrition, and School Failure* (New York: Harcourt Brace Jovanovich and Grune & Stratton, 1970), was consulted frequently in this and subsequent chapters. Chapter 8, pp. 177-220, is on "Nutrition, Growth, and Development."

Good discussions of fats are in Henrietta Fleck, *Introduction to Nutrition* (New York: Macmillan, 1971; 2nd ed.), pp. 49-56, and Sir Stanley Davidson, R. Passmore, and J.F. Brock, *Human Nutrition and Dietetics* (Baltimore: Williams & Wilkins, 1972; 5th ed.), pp. 62-77. In fact, both books are extremely valuable for almost any aspect of nutritional information. A good survey of the B vitamins is in Fleck's chapters 11 and 12.

Conclusions of the Longevity Foundation of America are in Jon N. Leonard, Jack L. Hofer, and Nathan Pritikin, *Live Longer Now* (New York: Grosset & Dunlap, 1974). See especially pp. 17-63. The Anderson–Herman findings are in James W. Anderson and Robert H. Herman, "Effects of Carbohydrate Restriction on Glucose Tolerance of Normal Men and Reactive Hypoglycemic Patients." *American Journal of Clinical Nutrition* vol. 28, no. 7 (July 1975), pp. 748-55.

Information on vitamin A overdose is in Norman J. Siegel and Thomas J. Spackman, "Chronic Hypervitaminosis A With

Intracranal Hypertension and Low Cerebrospinal Fluid Concentration of Protein," *Clinical Pediatrics* vol. 11, no. 10 (October, 1972), pp. 580–84.

In addition to general works pertinent to the B vitamins, a clinical study on pyridoxine is John M. Ellis and James Presley, *Vitamin B6: The Doctor's Report* (New York: Harper & Row, 1973). Roger Williams' experiments with rats involving pantothenic acid and longevity are described in his *Nutrition Against Disease: Environmental Prevention* (New York: Pitman Publishing, 1971). See also E. P. Ralli and M. E. Dumm, "Relation of Pantothenic Acid to Adrenal Cortical Function," *Vitamins and Hormones* vol. 11 (1953), p. 135 ff., and S. Maurer and L. S. Tsai, "Vitamin B Deficiency and Learning Ability," *Journal of Comparative Psychology* vol. 11, no. 1 (Oct., 1930), pp. 51–62.

Data on vitamin C are in Robert E. Hodges, "The Effect of Stress on Ascorbic Acid Metabolism in Man," *Nutrition Today* vol. 5, no. 1 (Spring, 1970), pp. 11–12; Linus Pauling, *Vitamin C and the Common Cold* (San Francisco: W. H. Freeman, 1970); Irwin Stone, *The Healing Factor: "Vitamin C" Against Disease* (New York: Grosset & Dunlap, 1972); and Frederick R. Klenner, "Observations on the Dose and Administration of Ascorbic Acid When Employed Beyond the Range of a Vitamin in Human Pathology," *Journal of Applied Nutrition* vol. 23, nos. 3 & 4 (Winter, 1971), pp. 61–88.

One of the most valuable books on trace minerals is Henry A. Schroeder, *The Trace Elements and Man; Some Positive and Negative Aspects* (Old Greenwich, Conn.: Devin-Adair Co., 1973). The essential role of one trace mineral is discussed in D. M. Hadjimarkos and Thomas R. Shearer, "Selenium in Mature Human Milk." *American Journal of Clinical Nutrition* vol. 26, no. 6 (June, 1973), pp. 583–85. A theory and compilation of evidence as to the crucial relationship of two trace minerals are in Leslie M. Klevay, "Coronary Heart Disease: The Zinc/Copper Hypothesis," *American Journal of Clinical Nutrition* vol. 28 (July, 1975), pp. 764–74.

An interesting validation of vitamin E is in Emanuel Cheraskin and W. Marshall Ringsdorf, Jr., *Predictive Medicine:*

A Study in Strategy (Mountain View, Calif.: Pacific Press Publishing Association, 1973), pp. 152–56.

An extensive discussion of natural foods is in Joe D. Nichols and James Presley, *Please, Doctor, Do Something!* (Old Greenwich, Conn.: Devin-Adair Co., 1972).

3. The Malnutrition of Affluence

A general work on infancy is Williams McKim Marriott and P.C. Jeans, *Infant Nutrition: A Textbook of Infant Feeding for Students and Practitioners of Medicine* (St. Louis: C. V. Mosby Co., 1941; 3rd ed.).

Early work on the dangers of milk and low protein in the preschool child appeared in Harold D. Lynch and William D. Snively, Jr., "Hypoproteinosis of Childhood," *Journal of the American Medical Association* vol. 147 (Sept. 8, 1951), pp. 115–19, and "Is Your Child Underprivileged?" *National Parent-Teacher* (December, 1951). See also Julian P. Price and Walter Moore Hart, "Malnutrition and Anemia in Young Children," *JAMA* vol. 48, no. 1 (Jan. 5, 1952), and Eugene Rosamund, "Further Observations on the Evils of Too Much Milk," *Southern Medical Journal* vol. 28 (Jan., 1935), pp. 46–47.

Information regarding parental concept of a "good breakfast" in the Arlington, Texas, study came from a personal communication, Nancy Bower.

The pig experiments on carbohydrates' effects in low-protein diet are in B. S. Platt, G. Pampiglione, and R. J. C. Stewart, "Experimental Protein-Calorie Deficiency: Clinical, Electroencephalographic and Neuropathological Changes in Pigs," *Developmental Medicine and Child Neurology* vol. 7 (1965), pp. 9–26.

Yudkin's testimony is in *Hearings Before the Select Committee on Nutrition and Human Needs, United States Senate, 93rd Congress, 1st Session: Nutrition and Disease—1973* (Washington: U.S. Government Printing Office, 1973), Part 2—Sugar in Diet, Diabetes, and Heart Disease (Series 73/ND2), p. 224 ff. See also John Yudkin, *Sweet and Dangerous* (New York: Peter Wyden, 1972), especially ch. 14, and T. L. Cleave, G. D. Campbell and N. S. Painter, *Diabetes, Coronary Thrombosis, and the Saccharine Disease* (Bristol, England: John Wright & Sons, 1969; 2nd ed.).

Sorbitol is discussed in Davidson, Passmore, and Brock, *Human Nutrition and Dietetics* (cited), pp. 44, 424.

The Banting quotation is from Sam Roberts, *Exhaustion: Diagnosis and Treatment, A New Approach to the Treatment of Allergy* (Emmaus, Pa.: Rodale Books, 1967), p. 59.

The impact of TV on children's nutrition is depicted in Joan Gussow, "It Makes Even Milk a Dessert": A Report on the Counter-nutritional Messages of Children's Television Advertising, *Clinical Pediatrics* vol. 12, no. 2 (Feb., 1973), pp. 68–71, and "Childrens TV: Sugar Makes Cents," *News & Comments: American Academy of Pediatrics* vol. 24, no. 6 (July, 1973), pp. 10–12.

The Platt and Chaplin experiments on the persistence of sugar preference are cited in Herbert G. Birch and Joan Dye Gussow, *Disadvantaged Children: Health, Nutrition, and School Failure* (New York: Harcourt Brace Jovanovich/Grune & Stratton, 1970), p. 149. See also K. Duncker, "Experimental Modification of Children's Food Preferences Through Social Suggestion," *Journal of Abnormal Social Psychology* vol. 33 (1938), pp. 489–507.

Excellent articles on sugar are Daniel Henninger, "Soured on Sugar," *National Observer* (Oct. 6, 1973), and Jane Ogle, "Killer on the Breakfast Table?" *Harper's Bazaar* (Oct., 1973), pp. 150–51, 168.

4. Building Resistance Against Illness

The Cheraskin-Ringsdorf material is from their *Predictive Medicine*, cited earlier, pp. 41, 174–75.

A good discussion of nutrition during pregnancy is in Roger J. Williams, *Nutrition Against Disease*, already cited, pp. 51–66. A journalistic account of the Mexico City conference and breast-feeding is in "Bottle-Fed Babies Doomed to Obesity, Scientists Report," *Dallas Times/Herald* (circa Sept. 14, 1972). The comparison of breast-fed babies with those on formulas was given in Carolyn Hoefer and Mattie Crumpton Hardy, "Later Development of Breast Fed and Artificially Fed Infants: Comparison of Physical and Mental Growth," *Journal of the*

American Medical Association vol. 92, no. 8 (1929), pp. 615–19.

For the classical work on stress, see Hans Selye, *The Stress of Life* (New York: McGraw Hill, 1956). For his observations on the stress of illness and food in hospitals, see Hans Selye, "On Just Being Sick," *Nutrition Today* vol. 5, no. 1 (Spring, 1970), pp. 2–10.

Material on phagocytic index and sugar comes from "Phagocytic Activity Depressed If Patient Is in Poor Condition," *Pediatric News* (Oct., 1973); Emanuel Cheraskin lecture, Dallas County (Texas) Dental Society, Dallas, Sept. 10, 1972 (tape recording); and Albert Sanchez, J. L. Reeser, H. S. Lau, P. Y. Yahiku, R. E. Willard, P. J. McMillan, S. Y. Cho, A. R. Magie, and U. D. Register, "Role of Sugars in Human Neutrophilic Phagocytosis," *American Journal of Clinical Nutrition* 26 (Nov., 1973), pp. 1180–1184.

The malnutrition-illness cycle is discussed in Birch and Gussow's *Disadvantaged Children*, p. 179 ff.

The impact of sucrose on vitamin C is in A. T. S. H. Setyaadmadja, E. Cheraskin, and W. M. Ringsdorf, Jr., "Ascorbic Acid and Carbohydrate Metabolism. II. Effect of Supervised Sucrose Drinks Upon Two-Hour Postprandial Blood Glucose in Terms of Vitamin C State," *The Lancet* vol. 87 (1967), pp. 18–21.

Discussion of the Peruvian children recovering from malnutrition is in George G. Graham and Blanca T. Adrianzen, "Late 'Catch-up' Growth After Severe Infantile Malnutrition," *Johns Hopkins Medical Journal* vol. 131 (1972), pp. 204–11. See also reports of a similar conclusion by Harvard Medical School investigators in "Effects of Malnutrition Appear Reversible," *Medical Tribune* (July 4, 1973), p. 19.

5. *"Why Doesn't He Behave?"*

For details on rapid blood sugar drop, see Guy Lacy Schless, "Ward Round: Diabetes," *British Journal of Hospital Medicine* (Dec., 1968), pp. 389–97. On symptoms of low blood sugar, see Gilles Lortie and Dean M. Laird, "Hypoglycemia Simulating Psychoses," *New England Journal of Medicine* vol. 256, no. 25 (June 20, 1957), pp. 1190–1192.

E. Cheraskin, W.M. Ringsdorf, Jr., and J. W. Clark, *Diet and Disease* (Emmaus, Pa.: Rodale Books, 1968), pp. 186–207, discusses how diet affects behavior and psychological reactions. The Brožek quotation is from Josef Brožek, "Experimental Studies on the Impact of Deficient Diet on Behavior," *Borden's Review of Nutritional Research* vol. 20, no. 6 (Nov.-Dec., 1959), pp. 75–88.

The Massler and Wood material on thumbsucking is from their article in *Journal of Dentistry of Children* vol. 16 (1949), pp. 1–9.

Classic studies on hypoglycemia are E. M. Abrahamson and A. W. Pezet, *Body, Mind, and Sugar* (New York: Holt, Rinehart, and Winston, 1951; paperback, Pyramid Books, 1971); and Carlton Fredericks and Herman Goodman, *Low Blood Sugar and You* (New York: Constellation International, 1969). See also S. A. Mann, "Blood-Sugar Studies in Mental Disorders," *Journal of Mental Science* vol. 71, no. 294 (July, 1925), pp. 443–73; J. I. Rodale, *Natural Health, Sugar, and the Criminal Mind* (New York: Pyramid Books, 1968); and Carlson Wade, "How Nutrition May Tame Violence," *Let's Live* (Sept., 1972), p. 28 ff.

One of the most valuable and thorough technical publications on megavitamin therapy and schizophrenia is David Hawkins and Linus Pauling, editors, *Orthomolecular Psychiatry: Treatment of Schizophrenia* (San Francisco: W. H. Freeman & Co., 1973). Numerous articles have been published in the popular health magazine, *Prevention,* from time to time. One of the best series of articles in the daily press was by Lynn Lilliston in the *Los Angeles Times,* beginning Nov. 26, 1972.

For a different approach to vitamin therapy, see George Watson, *Nutrition and Your Mind: The Psychochemical Response* (New York: Harper & Row, 1972). Its appendix, pp. 149–70, contains his technical, more specific article, "Differences in Intermediate Metabolism in Mental Illness," which originally appeared in *Psychological Reports* vol. 17 (1965), pp. 563–82.

Rimland's views are in Bernard Rimland, "Freud Is Dead: New Directions in the Treatment of Mentally Ill Children," address in Distinguished Lectures in Special Education series, University of Southern California, Los Angeles, July 7, 1970 (reprint), and Bernard Rimland, "High-Dosage Levels of Certain Vitamins in the Treatment of Children With Severe Mental Disorders," in Hawkins and Pauling, eds. op. cit., pp. 513-39.

Other alternate approaches come from Marshall Mandell, personal communication to James Presley; Allan Cott, "Megavitamins: The Orthomolecular Approach to Behavioral Disorders and Learning Disabilities," *Academic Therapy* vol. 7, no. 3 (Spring, 1972), pp. 245-58. Silbergeld's tracing of hyperactivity to lead is in *Dallas Morning News* (Oct. 5, 1973) p. 17A.

Early material on the Feingold thesis came from personal communication, Ben F. Feingold to James Presley; Ben F. Feingold, "Food Additives and Child Development," editorial, *Hospital Practice*, October, 1973, pp. 11-12 ff; and Ben F. Feingold, "Adverse Reactions to Food Additives, With Special Reference to Hyperkinesis and Learning Difficulty (H-LD)," paper presented to Symposium on Food, The Royal Institution, London, 1973. The summary popular book is Ben F. Feingold, *Why Your Child Is Hyperactive* (New York: Random House, 1975).

On the "wild child" see Mark A. Stewart, "Hyperactive Children," *Scientific American* (April, 1970), pp. 94-98, and Samuel Bogoch and Jack Dreyfus, *The Blood Range of Use of Diphenylhydantoin: Bibliography and Review* (The Dreyfus Medical Foundation, 1970).

Serotonin is covered in John J. Miller, "Serotonin—Friend or Foe?" *Journal of Applied Nutrition* vol. 17, nos. 2, 3 (Nov., 1964); Hemmige N. Bhagavan, Mary Coleman, and David Baird Coursin, "The Effect of Pyridoxine Hydrochloride on Blood Serotonin and Pyridoxal Phosphate Contents in Hyperactive Children," *Pediatrics* vol. 55, no. 3 (March, 1975), pp. 437-41; and John D. Fernstrom and Richard J. Wurtman, "Nutrition and the Brain," *Scientific American* vol. 230 (1974), pp. 84-91.

The statistical study of 98 hyperactive children in my practice is in Ida B. Anderson, "An Investigation of Diet and Vitamin

Therapy As a Method of Treatment in Reduction of Hyperactivity," unpublished Ed. D. dissertation, University of Northern Colorado, Greeley, Colorado, 1975. See especially pp. 100–101.

6. Why Some Children Don't Learn

Works examined with profit include C. H. Delacato, *The Diagnosis and Treatment of Speech and Reading Problems* (Springfield, Ill.: Charles Thomas, 1965); E. B. LeWinn, *Human Neurological Organization* (Springfield, Ill.: Charles C. Thomas, 1969); J. W. Tintera, "The Hypoadrenocortical State and Its Management," *New York State Journal of Medicine*, vol. 55, no. 33 (July 1, 1955); Walter B. Cannon, *The Wisdom of the Body* (New York: W. W. Norton & Co., 1963); F. H. Netter, *Endocrine System and Selected Metabolic Diseases*, vol. 4 (CIBA Collection of Medical Illustration).

Hoffman's work is detailed in M.S. Hoffman, "Early Indications of Learning Problems," *Academic Therapy* vol. 7, no. 1 (Fall, 1971), pp. 23–35.

Vitamins and learning ability are discussed in Ruth F. Harrell, Ella R. Woodyard, and Arthur I. Gates, "The Influence of Vitamin Supplementation of the Diets of Pregnant and Lactating Women on the Intelligence of Their Offspring," *Metabolism* vol. 5 (1956), pp. 555–62, and Siegfried Maurer and Loh Seng Tsai, "Vitamin B Deficiency and Learning Disability," *Journal of Comparative Psychology* vol. 11; (Oct., 1931), pp. 51–62.

Material relating to nutrition and brain development is surveyed in Merril S. Read, "The Biological Bases: Malnutrition and Behavioral Development," in *Seventy-First Yearbook of the National Society for the Study of Education* (Chicago, Ill.: University of Chicago Press, 1972), Part II, pp. 55–70, and Delbert H. Dayton, "Early Malnutrition and Human Development, *Children* vol. 16, no. 6 (Nov.-Dec., 1969), pp. 211–17.

The Birch-Gussow material is in their *Disadvantaged Children*, pp. 209–12. The Kryston comments are from Leonard Kryston, lecture, Seminar Workshop in Orthomolecular and Metabolic Approach to Childhood Disease, sponsored by the New York Institute of Child Development (Jan. 29, 1972, New York) tape recording.

The Arlington study, "Evaluation Design Nutrition Project," was dated Nov. 3, 1972.

A review of caffein's effects upon children is in Hugh W.S. Powers, Jr., "Caffein, Behavior, and the Learning Disability Child," *Academic Therapy* vol. XI: 1 (Fall, 1975), pp. 5–19. Greden's study is in his "Caffein Effects May Mimic Anxiety Neurosis State," *Clinical Psychiatry News* vol. 2, no. 6 (June, 1974). Also see Michael F. Jacobson, *The Eater's Digest* (New York: Doubleday Anchor Books, 1973), pp. 89–93, for further insight into the dangers of caffein.

The teacher's view of changing student behavior is in "Teacher Quits Due to Heartsickness," *Dallas Morning News*, Sept. 14, 1973, in Alice Skelsey's column, "For Women Who Work," syndicated by Chicago *Tribune*-New York *News* Syndicate.

The junior high observation regarding the machines was made in a letter from Robert L. Palmer to Nancy Judy, Nov. 25, 1974.

7. *Making Household Pediatrics Work*

The study at Northwestern University regarding weight loss upon spreading food intake out is in Edgar S. Gordon, Marshall Goldberg, and Grace J. Chosy, "A New Concept in the Treatment of Obesity," *Journal of the AMA* vol. 186, no. 1 (Oct. 5, 1963), pp. 50–60.

On bacon see Michael F. Jacobson, *How Sodium Nitrite Can Affect Your Health: "Don't Bring Home the Bacon"* (Washington: Center for Science in the Public Interest, 1973), pp. 1–53.

On various aspects of practical application of this chapter, see Jane Kinderlehrer, *Confessions of a Sneaky Organic Cook, Or How to Make Your Family Healthy When They're Not Looking!* (Emmaus, Pa.: Rodale Press, 1971; paperback, New York: New American Library, 1972); Betty Peterkin, *Your Money's Worth in Foods* (Washington: Government Printing Office), U.S. Department of Agriculture Home and Garden Bulletin No. 183; and *Nutrition—Applied Personally* (La Habra, Calif.: International College of Applied Nutrition, 1973).

Appendix A

For pertinent data on homeostasis, see E. Cheraskin, W.M. Ringsdorf, Jr., and J.W. Clark, *Diet and Disease* (Emmaus, Pa.: Rodale Books, 1968), pp. 52–61, 73 ff., and E. Cheraskin and W. M. Ringsdorf, Jr., *Predictive Medicine: A Study in Strategy* (Mountain View, Calif.: Pacific Press Publishing Association, 1973), pp. 136–50.

APPENDIX A

The Homeostasis Test

Although in this book I have used the glucose tolerance test (GTT) as a major diagnostic tool, there is another method of testing how the body handles sugars. This is the *homeostasis* test, which is conducted differently from the GTT and which tests for slightly different substances.

In treating children, the five-hour glucose tolerance test has been found to be very effective; a major reason for this is that it more dramatically depicts how the child or youth is handling ingested sugar. It is what is called a provocative loading test, in that the child swallows a measured amount of glucose on an empty stomach; thereafter during the test his blood glucose levels are analyzed at regular intervals, at half-hour intervals at first and then at hourly points during the remainder of the period.

However, other physicians have found the homeostasis test to be very valuable; some, dealing with adult patients, prefer it to the GTT.

For this book, I have consulted with James R. Hill, M.D., a former president of the International Academy of Metabology who is an authority on both the GTT and the homeostasis test, regarding the technical differences between the two tests.

Dr. Hill has used both tests extensively and now prefers the homeostasis test. However, it must be remembered that Dr. Hill's patients are all adults, since he is a specialist in internal medicine, and as he points out, "Many of my patients have already seen ten physicians and two psychiatrists before they come to me." In other words, the patient is by then convinced that he is very ill; graphic demonstration of his blood sugar fluctuations is rarely necessary.

The readings on the two tests are different. For instance, on the GTT, following the Tintera standard, the ideal fasting level should be 110 milligrams percent, and the blood sugar level should return to this original figure two hours after the glucose loading. However, a healthy blood sugar level in the homeostasis test should always be between 75 and 85 milligrams percent. It should never deviate outside that range, neither higher nor lower.

On the surface, these two ideal blood sugar levels appear to be in conflict. However, the conflict is only apparent, because of the different factors that are measured in the blood.

As Dr. Hill points out, the Tintera ideal standard is based on the GTT using the Folin-Wu method, which tests for *all* sugars, not merely glucose. If the lab tests for all sugar substances, then it should reflect a higher figure. The homeostasis test, however, is the Cheraskin glucose oxidase test after Dr. Emanuel Cheraskin, which tests for "true sugar" or glucose only; therefore the reading is a lower figure. They are not testing for the same things.

An advantage of the homeostasis test is that the patient

eats his or her own diet during the test day and keeps a precise diet diary. The doctor then can correlate the particular values on the test with the particular food that was eaten. This may enable the doctor to pinpoint the precise food that is giving the patient trouble and therefore bring it to the patient's attention.

As Dr. Emanuel Cheraskin and associates point out in *Diet and Disease*, the body must remain in a homeostatic, or steady, state constantly for there to be a condition of health. Following this standard of homeostasis for blood sugar, it is important to remember that even slight deviations from the 75 to 85 milligrams percent homeostatic range also reflect deviations from health. Such slight deviations may indicate a relatively serious imbalance in the body's metabology.

During the homeostasis test, blood samples are drawn from the patient at two-hour intervals (instead of hourly as in the GTT), at 8:30 A.M., 10:30 P.M., 12:30 P.M., 2:30 P.M., and 4:30 P.M. The patient's food diary that day indicates the exact time at which food was taken and exactly what and how much was eaten or drunk.

With some patients, I have used both tests. The GTT was first used to diagnose the problem's severity; subsequently, the homeostasis test was used as a follow-up if the patient did not respond as expected.

Let me illustrate how these two tests are used, through the case of a patient whom I will call Stephanie. I will restrict this presentation to those aspects that are pertinent to this illustration.

Stephanie was nine years, nine months old. A poorly developed little girl, she had suffered growth failure, it seemed. Although she did well on much of her examination, she had a learning disability, having completed the third grade with low marks. She had indications of mild hyperactivity and although she was cheerful when she awoke in the mornings, she both walked and talked in her sleep at times.

Her diet was not nearly as bad as many patients described in this book, but she did drink caffein in the form of tea and may have been ingesting other deleterious foods. She had suffered allergies to eggs, milk, tuna, corn, and wheat in the past; at sixteen months of age, she had survived an episode of paint poisoning. (Therefore, the possibility of lead poisoning became a factor in the diagnosis.)

Given a five-hour GTT, an erratic pattern resulted in her blood sugar curve that is shown in Figure A-1.

Over an extended period of time, Stephanie improved in many respects, including in learning and behavior. However, she remained markedly underdeveloped at age thirteen, with no menarche (beginning of menstruation). Her central nervous system seemed to be in excellent condition and she was making good progress in her special training for the learning disability.

At this point she was administered the homeostasis test. (See Figure A–2.) Her readings were:

8:30 A.M.	62
10:30 A.M.	62
12:30 P.M.	77
2:30 P.M.	100
4:30 P.M.	89

Only once was her reading within the 75 to 85 range that is homeostatic. She started out with too little glucose in her blood. By afternoon it was too high; then it began to fall.

Let us look at what Stephanie was eating that day and how it may have affected her blood sugar levels. At 7:30 A.M. she ate a half-cup of a so-called sugarless jello. Although her mother didn't realize it, it contained sorbitol, which can do the same thing to the patient that

Figure A-1. Stephanie's Glucose Tolerance Test

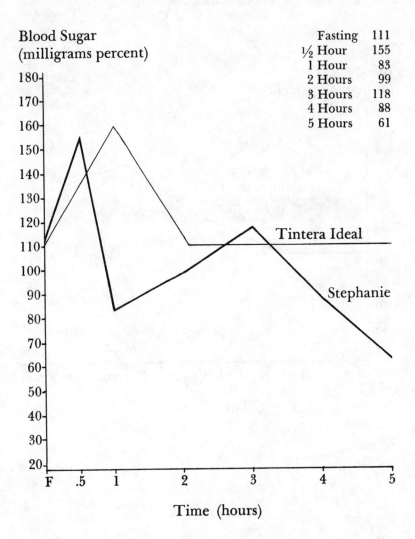

Blood Sugar
(milligrams percent)

Fasting	111
½ Hour	155
1 Hour	83
2 Hours	99
3 Hours	118
4 Hours	88
5 Hours	61

Tintera Ideal

Stephanie

Time (hours)

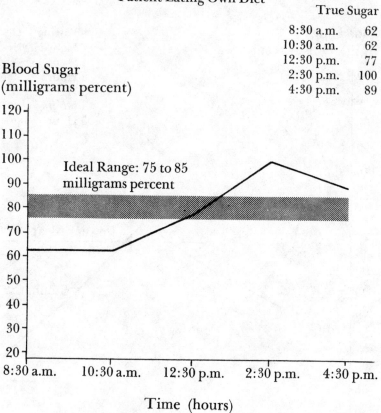

Figure A-2. Stephanie's Homeostasia Blood Sugar Curve

Patient Eating Own Diet

	True Sugar
8:30 a.m.	62
10:30 a.m.	62
12:30 p.m.	77
2:30 p.m.	100
4:30 p.m.	89

Blood Sugar
(milligrams percent)

Ideal Range: 75 to 85
milligrams percent

Time (hours)

sucrose does. At 9 A.M. she took four ounces of tomato juice, a slice of ham, and half a pecan waffle. (Depending on the type of flour that went into the waffle and whether syrup was used with it, this may also have been a suspect food.)

At 11:30 A.M. she had a six-ounce bottle of Diet Dr. Pepper. The mother thought she was avoiding trouble with this because it was a "diet," presumably sugarless, drink. However, it did have caffein in it; all dark-colored beverages should be avoided for this reason, if for no other.

The blood sugar started climbing at this point. The cola drink had picked Stephanie up; probably her fatigue had made her want it in the first place. But the cola picked her up too much, beyond the homeostatic range.

At 1 P.M., following her third blood sample, she lunched on ¼ cup of green beans, ¼ cup of mashed potatoes, a slice of roast beef, one cube of watermelon, and a half-pint of milk. By 2:30 P.M. her blood sugar had reached its peak in the test; thereafter it began declining back toward the homeostatic ideal. The meal could probably be credited with her blood sugar moving back toward a more desirable level. (It usually takes about two hours for the impact of solid food to be made on the blood sugar.) But by 4:30 P.M. when the last blood sample was drawn, she still had not returned to the 75–85 range.

After the test was over that day, Stephanie ate a chicken thigh at 4:45 P.M. and at 5:30 P.M. she had six ounces more of the diet drink—which probably pushed up her sagging blood sugar, albeit too high. Her dinner consisted of ¼ cup of french fries, half a hamburger, and six ounces more of the diet (caffeinated) drink.

By studying all these factors and the blood sugar graph, it was easy to show Stephanie and her mother what was still being done wrong in the nutritional program. Her mother had not understood that the "diet" drink was caffeinated. Nor did she realize that the "sugarless" jello contained sorbitol, which could be as suspicious as sucrose. But by recognizing these dietary indiscretions and relating them to Stephanie's blood sugar curve, the mother was able to reorganize her daughter's eating habits more in line with what she *thought* she had been getting. Eliminating these hitherto unrecognized factors in the diet would not necessarily solve all of Stephanie's medical problems, but it would be another step in the right direction.

APPENDIX B

Foods High In Essential Nutrients

Foods are listed in approximate amounts supplied by average servings, highest first and decreasing down. (These tables are reprinted by permission of Dietronics, Box 35, Northridge, California 91324.)

PROTEIN	VITAMIN C	THREONINE
Eggs	Citrus	(essential amino
Milk, cheese	Fresh fruits	acid)
Fish	Berries	Fish
Chicken	Broccoli	Beef
Beef	Tomatoes	Organ meats
Pork	Green leafy	Eggs
Soybeans	vegetables	Shellfish
Beans, peas	Baked potatoes	Soya
Nuts	Turnips	Liver
Corn		

FATS
Margarine
Butter
Peanut butter
Salad oils
Cream, cheese
Bacon, pork
Beef
Fish

POLYUN-SATURATED FATTY ACIDS
Margarine from
    safflower, corn,
    soy (non
    hydrogenated)
Corn oil (35%)
Safflower oil (70%)
Peanut oil (28%)
Soybean oil (50%)
Cottonseed oil (50%)
Lard (10%)

VITAMIN A
Carrots
Green leafy
    vegetables
Butter
Whole milk
Liver
Fish

VITAMIN B$_1$
Liver
Pork
Yeast
Organ meats
Whole grains
Bread
Wheat germ
Peanuts

VITAMIN E
Margarine
Oil salad dressing
Vegetable oils
Eggs
Cereal germ

TRYPTOPHANE
(essential amino
    acid)
Soy milk
Fish
Beef
Soy flour
Organ meats
Shellfish
Eggs

PHENYLALANINE
(essential amino
    acid)
Beef
Fish
Eggs
Whole Wheat
Shellfish
Organ meats
Soya
Milk

LEUCINE (essential amino acid)
Beef
Fish
Organ meats
Eggs
Soya
Shellfish
Whole wheat
Milk
Liver

IODINE
Iodized salt
Shellfish
Ocean fish
Bacon

CALCIUM
Cheese
Milk
Bread
Nuts
Legumes
Green leafy
    vegetables

IRON
Liver
Organ meats
Eggs
Legumes
Green leafy
    vegetables
Oysters

POTASSIUM
Green leafy
    vegetables
Legumes
Nuts
Cocoa
Vegetable juices

MAGNESIUM
Soya flour
Whole wheat
Oatmeal
Peas
Brown rice
Whole corn
Beans
Nuts

218

VITAMIN B$_2$
Eggs
Liver
Yeast
Milk
Whole grains
Bread
Wheat germ

NIACIN
Yeast
Liver
Wheat bran
Peanuts
Beans

PANTOTHENIC ACID
Liver
Organ meats
Eggs
Yeast
Wheat bran
Legumes
Cereals

VITAMIN B$_6$
Wheat germ
Kidney
Liver
Ham
Organ meats
Legumes
Peanuts

VITAMIN B$_{12}$
Liver
Organ meats
Oysters
Salmon
Eggs
Beef

ISO-LEUCINE
(essential amino acid)
Fish
Beef
Organ meats
Eggs
Shellfish
Whole wheat
Soya
Milk

LYSINE (essential amino acid)
Fish
Beef
Organ meats
Shellfish
Eggs
Soya
Milk
Liver

VALINE (essential amino acid)
Beef
Fish
Organ meats
Eggs
Soya
Milk
Whole wheat
Liver

METHIONINE
(essential amino acid)
Fish
Beef
Shellfish
Eggs
Milk
Liver
Whole wheat
Cheese

PHOSPHORUS
Highest dietary sources include protein foods such as
Soya flour
Whole wheat
Oatmeal
Peas
Brown rice
Whole corn
Beans
Nuts

SODIUM
The greatest portion of sodium is provided by table salt and salt used in cooking. Foods high in sodium include:
Dried beef
Ham
Canned corned beef
Bacon
Wheat breads
Salted crackers
Flaked breakfast cereals
Olives
Cheese
Butter
Margarine
Sausage
Dried fish
Canned vegetables
Shellfish and salt water fish
Raw celery

Refs: — Wahl & Goodhart, Modern Nutrition in Health & Disease, Lea & Febiger 1964;—Heinz Handbook of Nutrition;—Bicknell & Prescott, The Vitamins in Medicine, 3rd Ed. Heinemann, 1953;—U.S. Dept. Agriculture Food Tables;—Bowes & Church, Food Values, J.B. Lippincott 10th Ed.;—Kleiner & Orden, Biochemistry, 7th Ed. C.V. Mosby Co., 1966.

Hidden Sugars
in Foods

The patient often says, "Doctor, I don't eat sugar!" Here are the approximate amounts of refined sugar hidden in common foods—about which the patient is usually unaware.

FOOD ITEM	PORTION SIZE	APPROXIMATE SUGAR CONTENT (TEASPOONSFULS) GRANULATED SUGAR
Beverages		
Cola drinks	1 (6 oz. bottle or glass)	4⅓
Cordials	1 (¾ oz. glass)	1½
Ginger ale	6 oz.	3⅓
Hi-ball	1 (6 oz. glass)	2½
Orangeade	1 (8 oz. glass)	5

FOOD ITEM	PORTION SIZE	APPROXIMATE SUGAR CONTENT (TEASPOONSFULS) GRANULATED SUGAR
Root beer	1 (10 oz. bottle)	4½
Seven-Up	1 (6 oz. bottle or glass)	3¾
Soda	1 (8 oz. bottle)	5
Sweet cider	1 cup	4½
Whiskey sour	1 (3 oz. glass)	1½

Jams and Jellies

Apple butter	1 tbsp.	1
Jelly	1 tbsp.	4-6
Orange marmalade	1 tbsp.	4-6
Peach butter	1 tbsp.	1
Strawberry jam	1 tbsp.	4

Cakes and Cookies

Angel food	1 (4 oz. piece)	7
Apple sauce cake	1 (4 oz. piece)	5½
Banana cake	1 (2 oz. piece)	2
Cheese cake	1 (4 oz. piece)	2
Chocolate cake (plain)	1 (4 oz. piece)	6
Chocolate cake (iced)	1 (4 oz. piece)	10
Coffee cake	1 (4 oz. piece)	4½
Cup cake (iced)	1	6
Fruit cake	1 (4 oz. piece)	5
Jelly-roll	1 (2 oz. piece)	2½
Orange cake	1 (4 oz. piece)	4
Pound cake	1 (4 oz. piece)	5

FOOD ITEM	PORTION SIZE	APPROXIMATE SUGAR CONTENT (TEASPOONSFULS) GRANULATED SUGAR
Sponge cake	1 (1 oz. piece)	2
Strawberry short cake	1 serving	4
Brownies (unfrosted)	1 (¾ oz.)	3
Molasses cookies	1	2
Chocolate cookies	1	1½
Fig newtons	1	5
Ginger snaps	1	3
Macaroons	1	6
Nut cookies	1	1½
Oatmeal cookies	1	2
Sugar cookies	1	1½
Chocolate eclair	1	7
Cream puff	1	2
Donut (plain)	1	3
Donut (glazed)	1	6
Snail	1 (4 oz. piece)	4½

Candies

Average chocolate milk bar (example: Hershey bar)	1 (1½ oz.)	2½
Chewing gum	1 stick	½
Chocolate cream	1 piece	2
Butterscotch chew	1 piece	1
Chocolate mints	1 piece	2
Fudge	1 oz. square	4½

FOOD ITEM	PORTION SIZE	APPROXIMATE SUGAR CONTENT (TEASPOONSFULS) GRANULATED SUGAR
Gum drop	1	2
Hard candy	4 oz.	20
Lifesavers	1	⅓
Peanut brittle	1 oz.	3½
Marshmallow	1	1½

Canned Fruits and Juices

Raisins	¼ cup	4
Currants, dried	1 tbsp.	4
Persimmons, fresh	¼ cup	7
Fruit cocktail	½ cup scant	5
Orange juice	½ cup scant	2
Pineapple juice (unsweetened)	½ cup scant	2-3/5
Grapejuice (commercial)	½ cup scant	3⅔
Rhubarb, stewed	½ cup sweetened	8
Canned apricots	4 halves & 1 T syrup	3½
Applesauce (unsweetened)	½ cup scant	2
Canned fruit juices (sweetened)	½ cup	2
Prunes, stewed (sweetened)	4-5 med., 2 tsp. juice	8
Canned peaches	2 halves & 1 T syrup	3½
Prunes, dried	3-4 med.	4
Fruit salad	½ cup	3½
Apricots, dried	4-6 halves	4

224

FOOD ITEM	PORTION SIZE	APPROXIMATE SUGAR CONTENT (TEASPOONSFULS) GRANULATED SUGAR
Fruit syrup	2 T	2½
Dates, dried	3-4 stoned	4½
Stewed fruits	½ cup	2
Figs, dried	1½-2, small	4

Dairy Products

Ice cream	⅓ pt. (3½ oz.)	3½
Ice cream bar	1	1-7 depending on size
Cocoamalt, all milk	1 glass, 8 oz.	4 tsp
Ice cream cone	1	3½
Eggnog, all milk	1 glass, 8 oz.	4½ tsp
Ice cream soda	1	5
Cocoa, all milk	1 cup, 5 oz. milk	4 tsp
Ice cream sundae	1	7
Chocolate, all milk	1 cup, 5 oz. milk	6 tsp
Malted milk shake	1 (10 oz. glass)	5

Desserts, Miscellaneous

Apple cobbler	½ cup	3
Blueberry cobbler	½ cup	3
Custard	½ cup	2
French pastry	1 (4 oz. piece)	5
Jello	½ cup	4½
Gelatin	½ cup	4
Apple pie	1 slice (average)	7

FOOD ITEM	PORTION SIZE	APPROXIMATE SUGAR CONTENT (TEASPOONSFULS) GRANULATED SUGAR
Junket	⅛ quart	3
Apricot pie	1 slice	7
Berry pie	1 slice	10
Butterscotch pie	1 slice	4
Cherry pie	1 slice	10
Cream pie	1 slice	4
Custard pie	1 slice	10
Cocoanut pie	1 slice	10
Lemon pie	1 slice	7
Mince meat pie	1 slice	4
Peach pie	1 slice	7
Prune pie	1 slice	6
Pumpkin pie	1 slice	5
Rhubarb pie	1 slice	4
Raisin pie	1 slice	13
Banana pudding	½ cup	2
Bread pudding	½ cup	1½
Chocolate pudding	½ cup	4
Cornstarch pudding	½ cup	2½
Date pudding	½ cup	7
Fig pudding	½ cup	7
Grapenut pudding	½ cup	2
Plum pudding	½ cup	4
Rice pudding	½ cup	5
Tapioca pudding	½ cup	3
Berry tart	1	10
Blanc-mange	½ cup	5
Brown betty	½ cup	3
Plain pastry	1 (4 oz. piece)	3
Sherbet	½ cup	9

FOOD ITEM	PORTION SIZE	APPROXIMATE SUGAR CONTENT (TEASPOONSFULS) GRANULATED SUGAR
Syrups, Sugars and Icings		
Brown sugar	1 tbsp.	3 (actual sugar content)
Chocolate icing	1 oz.	5
Chocolate sauce	1 tbsp.	3½
Corn syrup	1 tbsp.	3 (actual sugar content)
Granulated sugar	1 tbsp.	3 (actual sugar content)
Honey	1 tbsp.	3 (actual sugar content)
Karo syrup	1 tbsp.	3 (actual sugar content)
Maple syrup	1 tbsp.	5 (actual sugar content)
Molasses	1 tbsp.	3½ (actual sugar content)
White icing	1 oz.	5

Acknowledgments

I would like to acknowledge the assistance of the following persons for the parts they played in helping make this book a reality:

James R. Hill, M.D., a fellow pioneer in the field of orthomolecular medicine, who has shared his encyclopedic knowledge with me; Mary S. Hoffman, M.D., whom I would emulate for her eagerness to help children in trouble; Mrs. Elinor Reinmiller, reference librarian at the University of Texas Southwestern Health and Science Center, Dallas; Bill Hanson of Dietronics for his cooperation in the use of his company's food tables; Mrs. Willa Powell and Mrs. Karen Whittle, office assistants who labored at the typewriter and put up with impulsive demands to type, copy, and mail material to my collaborator; and my many grateful nutritional patients for their warm friendship and encouragement.

Finally, I wish to thank the inspired doctors and

nutritionists, many of whom I have met and admired, who have all opened the door to the provocative world of orthomolecular therapy.

—Hugh Powers, M.D.

For assisting me in my work on this book I wish to acknowledge the following persons:

Mayo Drake, librarian at the Louisiana State University School of Medicine in Shreveport, and his staff, especially Kathy Corbell, Marilyn Miller, Jan Wiemann, and Gerald Stephans, whose assistance in securing copies of difficult-to-find medical articles was little short of Herculean; the staff at the Memorial Library, Texas Medical Association for obtaining research materials; Mrs. W.R. Capshaw, librarian at the Texarkana Public Library for obtaining interlibrary loans. Max Watson was helpful with food-pricing information.

I especially wish to single out two persons whose association during the writing of this book has been vital to its completion. Blanche C. Gregory, my literary agent and friend who has been a major factor in my career, should be placed on a pedestal for her tireless efforts. Jay Acton, while my editor at St. Martin's Press, displayed the perception, energy and searching analysis that made this a better book. I appreciate both of them. In addition, Joanne Michaels, also my editor at St. Martin's Press, contributed her skill and enthusiasm at the end in a way that would thrill any author.

Bonnie Ray Cadwell contributed information that led to my becoming acquainted with my now good friend, Dr. Hugh Powers. Frances Burton, my mother-in-law and valued friend, not only encouraged but gave of her time at crucial stages in the research and writing, as did my father, J. A. Presley. I am also grateful to Birdie Porter for her contributions and friendship. Dr. Gilbert McAllister and

Cora McAllister, my close friends since I was Gilbert's student in graduate school long ago, have constantly encouraged me.

Corbett Anderson prepared the blood sugar charts that appear in the book. Elizabeth Wright, once again, assisted in the typing of the completed manuscript, cheerfully though under pressure.

Finally, my wife, Fran, who has been a major source of encouragement during all of my books, improved this one with her perceptive editorial suggestions and contributed the title.

—James Presley